Reflective Practice of Counseling
and Psychotherapy in a Diverse Society

Jason D. Brown

Reflective Practice of Counseling and Psychotherapy in a Diverse Society

palgrave
macmillan

Jason D. Brown
Faculty of Education
Western University
London, Canada

ISBN 978-3-030-24507-8   ISBN 978-3-030-24505-4   (eBook)
https://doi.org/10.1007/978-3-030-24505-4

This Palgrave Macmillan imprint is published by the registered company Springer Nature Switzerland AG
The registered company address is: Gewerbestrasse 11, 6330 Cham, Switzerland

Preface

Reflective Practice of Counseling and Psychotherapy in a Diverse Society

This book is for anyone practicing psychotherapy or counseling. It is my hope that over time and accumulation of experience that the topics remain relevant and the questions, worth considering again at different points in one's career.

The humanity of our work is vital to its practice. In this way, reflective practice can serve as a helpful guide to self-monitoring and improvement. The topics herein place particular importance on the potential for our work to be therapeutic in ways that are also emancipatory, inclusive, and equitable. Social location and identity are fundamental topics to consider for working in a diverse society and across differences. The success of efforts that directly and indirectly challenge privilege are essential to improve access to opportunities that enhance mental health and address illness for all who experience social disadvantage. One way to move this idea forward is to locate oneself in the systemic oppression associated with identities and locations that we are each a part of.

My own journey with this started as a student in social work and the realization of the privilege I hold as a White European settler, who is cisgender, heterosexual, and without a visible disability. While those privileges did not prevent me from experiencing my own mental health challenges, they did provide me with opportunities and expectations that many others did not have. They also did, when I realized the extent of their influence, produce a large dose of guilt and shame which took several years for me to understand. I have come to realize that efforts to promote social change need to start with an understanding of history and my people's place within it, followed by personal acknowledgment and commitment followed by concrete action.

The chapters can be read in any sequence. Each can also stand on its own. Each is meant to be concise and offer questions for consideration. It is my belief that reflective practice is a personal journey. However, readers might find some questions useful for group discussion. The activity in Chapter 10 is the only group activity in the book and could be used at any point.

I would be pleased to hear your comments and feedback.

Sincerely

London, Canada   Jason D. Brown

CONTENTS

LIST OF FIGURES

LIST OF TABLES

CHAPTER 1

Reflective Practice Framework

Therapists' perceptions shape the goals, activities, and outcomes of counseling and psychotherapy (Mahalik, Worthington, & Crump, 1999; Strupp, 1980). Reflective practice (RP) focuses on what professionals believe and value. It targets what is taken for granted. It invites professionals to challenge their assumptions. RP is the personal experience of meaning-making for self-awareness, cultural sensitivity, enhancement of the therapeutic relationship, as well as personal, professional, and social change.

WHAT IS REFLECTIVE PRACTICE?

RP is a process for professional and personal self-improvement.
RP includes what happened, why it happened, and how it happened.
RP explores processes occurring throughout and following an experience.
RP is a way of making meaning about why we do what we do.

WHAT IS NOT REFLECTIVE PRACTICE?

RP is not an identity, status (professional high ground), or achievement.
RP is not prescriptive, punitive, or uniform.
RP is not for personal therapy.
RP is not for guilt release.

© The Author(s) 2019   1
J. D. Brown, *Reflective Practice of Counseling and Psychotherapy in a Diverse Society*, https://doi.org/10.1007/978-3-030-24505-4_1

WHY DOES REFLECTIVE PRACTICE MATTER?

RP is a professional resource.
RP is a way to improve skill and effectiveness.
RP is a way to enhance cultural competence, the therapeutic relationship, use of emotion, and self-care.

I (JB) was practicing in a medium-sized city's downtown core counseling men who were released from institutions living in the community. As a professional corrections employee, it was an ethical responsibility to protect the public. I also felt it was necessary to connect with clients to understand the issues that led to incarceration. I some ways, such as their experience of being incarcerated for months to years, I had no point of reference and felt worlds apart. In other ways, I felt separated by only bad luck and some poor decisions. The struggles I had were about fairness, responsibility, and change. These were fundamental personal values tested by new professional experiences. For example, are trials, sentences as well as incarceration, and release applied fairly? Does responsibility for illicit behavior exist solely within the individual? If such behavior is in any way socially influenced, how much personal change is possible?

> Take a few minutes to consider the many values listed below and check those that matter most to you. Once you have done that, check to see if they can be grouped and ranked in order of importance.

Acceptance	Accomplishment	Accountability	Accuracy
Achievement	Adaptability	Adventure	Agility
Alertness	Altruism	Ambition	Amusement
Assertiveness	Attentive	Audacity	Authenticity
Authority	Autonomy	Awareness	Balance
Beauty	Belonging	Best	Boldness
Bravery	Brilliance	Calm	Candor
Capable	Careful	Certainty	Challenge
Charity	Cheerfulness	Citizenship	Cleanliness
Clear	Clever	Comfort	Commitment
Common sense	Communication	Community	Compassion
Competence	Competition	Concentration	Confidence
Connection	Consciousness	Consistency	Contentment
Contribution	Control	Conviction	Cooperation
Correctness	Courage	Courtesy	Creativity
Credibility	Curiosity	Decisiveness	Dedication
Dependability	Determination	Development	Devotion
Dignity	Discipline	Discovery	Discretion

Diversity	Drive	Duty	Dynamism
Economy	Effectiveness	Efficiency	Elegance
Empathy	Empower	Endurance	Energy
Enjoyment	Enthusiasm	Entrepreneurship	Equality
Equity	Ethical	Excellence	Excitement
Experience	Expertise	Exploration	Expressive
Fairness	Faith	Fame	Family
Fearless	Feelings	Ferocious	Fidelity
Fitness	Fluency	Focus	Foresight
Fortitude	Freedom	Friendship	Fun
Generosity	Genius	Giving	Goodness
Grace	Gratitude	Greatness	Growth
Happiness	Hard work	Harmony	Health
Helping	Holiness	Honesty	Honor
Hope	Humility	Humor	Imagination
Improvement	Independence	Individuality	Ingenuity
Innovation	Inquisitive	Insightful	Inspiring
Integrity	Intelligence	Intensity	Intuition
Irreverent	Joy	Justice	Kindness
Knowledge	Lawful	Leadership	Learning
Legacy	Leisure	Liberty	Logic
Love	Loyalty	Mastery	Maturity
Meaning	Merit	Moderation	Motivation
Nature	Obedience	Openness	Optimism
Order	Organization	Originality	Partnership
Passion	Patience	Patriotism	Peace
Perfection	Performance	Persistence	Piety
Playfulness	Poise	Positivity	Potential
Power	Practicality	Preparedness	Present
Prestige	Productivity	Professionalism	Prosperity
Prudence	Purpose	Quality	Realistic
Reason	Recognition	Recreation	Reflective
Relationship	Reliability	Resourcefulness	Respect
Responsibility	Restraint	Results	Reverence
Rigor	Risk	Satisfaction	Security
Self-actualization	Self-control	Self-reliance	Selfless
Sensitivity	Serenity	Service	Sharing
Shrewdness	Significance	Silence	Simplicity
Sincerity	Skill	Smart	Solitude
Soundness	Speed	Spirit	Spirituality
Spontaneous	Stability	Status	Stewardship
Strategic	Strength	Structure	Success
Support	Surprise	Sustainability	Talent
Teamwork	Temperance	Thankful	Thorough
Thoughtful	Timeliness	Tolerance	Toughness
Traditional	Tranquility	Transparency	Trust
Truth	Understanding	Uniqueness	Unity
Usefulness	Valor	Variety	Victory
Vigor	Vision	Vitality	Wealth
Welcoming	Winning	Wisdom	Wonder

PERSONAL VALUES AND REFLEXIVITY

The values we hold connect with our experience. They are at the center of RP. As you work through this text, return periodically to the values you identified and check their applicability to the topics as well as which are the most and least salient.

Reflexivity is considering self in context. It has been defined as "regular exercise of the mental ability, shared by all normal people, to consider themselves in relation to their (social) contexts and vice versa" (Donati & Archer, 2015, p. 62). It is an "internal conversation" Archer (2007) but oriented toward action. It includes professional self-awareness and the need to go beyond individual work to account for the impact of culture and social structure.

Ontology is the study of being. Assumptions are realism and relativism. Relativism holds that reality is existence constructed by perception. Realism holds that reality is existence independent of perception. Critical realism is a combination: some independent reality exists, but our perceptions are constructed. Dialectical Critical Realism holds that values underlie perceptions and that different perceptions of reality can exist simultaneously (Bagley, Abubaker, & Sawyerr, 2018).

Epistemology is the study of knowledge. Four sources include intuitive, authoritative, logical, and empirical. Intuitive is our gut or the values and specific beliefs we hold. Authoritative is from another source, and its weight rests on the credibility of the source. Logical knowledge is the rational connection between what is known and what is new. Empirical is based on observable and objective sources.

Reflexivity in the context of professional practice, "is aimed at problem-solving, building understanding from, and about, practice situations, the use of self, and, for improving and learning from practice" (Watts, 2019). It is rooted in our values and includes our beliefs about what is real as well as how we gain knowledge.

CRITICAL REFLECTION

Critical reflection is a way of making meaning of social, political, and economic conditions one experiences. It has the potential to change professional practice in counseling and psychotherapy (Butani, Blankenburg, & Long, 2013). Different traditions include interpretation, explanation, and critique (Hodgson & Watts, 2017, p. 238).

Critique is comparing what is to what is desirable. Interpretation is used to understand when new information occurs. An explanation is a detailed accounting of the relationship between phenomena. Critical reflection is used to describe a process of giving voice and meaning to experience and creates an acknowledgment of multiple ways of knowing (Fook, 2002).

REFLECTIVE PRACTICE

RP is a critical reflection for professional purposes. As such, it includes assumptions about what reality is and how it relates to other knowledge. RP involves the comparison of what is perceived relative to an ideal. RP may involve reflection in action, reflection on action, as well as the reflection of impact on others (Fisher, Chew, & Leow, 2015). It focuses on what we recognize, consider and do in the contexts within which we function (Napier & Fook, 2001; Finlayson, 2015; Fisher et al., 2015; Sandeen, Moore, & Swanda, 2018).

Approaches to Reflective Practice

Habermas (1972) describes reflection as a cognitive process for commonly used categories of experience. These categories include work, interaction, and power (Mezirow, 1981; Taylor, 2004), and are known as technical, practical, and emancipatory reflection, respectively.

Technical reflection is based on measurable qualities evaluated via the scientific method. The knowledge can be applied to similar circumstances to predict outcomes. This is useful for therapeutic practice and developing competence in specific tasks. It provides a basis for evidence-informed practice. It allows for the testing of existing practices to determine effectiveness.

Practical reflection is based on interpersonal interactions, norms, and social expectations understood through personal experience. Knowledge is developed over time. It is transmitted through language and filtered through what people think, feel, and do in context. The description of experience can further detail and organize what transpired in such a way that it becomes useful for others to integrate into their practice.

Emancipatory reflection utilizes the processes of interpretation in practical reflection but views social roles as transient or fluid.

Assumptions about what should be are questioned in light of the limiting effect of existing practices. It includes the awareness "of how an ideology reflects and distorts moral, social and political reality and what material and psychological factors influence and sustain the false consciousness which it represents —especially reified powers of domination" (Mezirow, 1981, p. 145). It includes deconstructing and confronting, as well as reconstructing and transforming personal, historical, social, political, and economic forces that affect one's practice (Taylor, 2017).

WHY USE REFLECTIVE PRACTICE?

Pollard (2002) notes that the distinction made by Dewey in *How We Think* (1933) between routinized and reflective learning is "fundamental to the conception of professional development" (p. 4). Reflective learning and practice embraces uncertainty and defies pressure for quick decision-making. Its practitioners tolerate a lack of clarity and surety and consider relevant factors commensurate with the potential impact. Without reflective practice, professionals may "cultivate an over-positive and dogmatic habit of mind or feel perhaps that a condition of doubt will be regarded as evidence of mental inferiority" (Dewey, p. 124) in Galea (2012). Reflective practice is increasingly recognized and incorporated into professional counseling and psychotherapy training (Mann, Gordon, & MacLeod 2009). It is essential for ethical practice and cultural competence as well as sound therapeutic judgment.

Ethical Practice

Professionals providing counseling and psychotherapy are required, as authorized members of their professions, to follow ethical principles and standards of practice. In psychology, for example, the American Psychological Association and Canadian Psychological Association have Ethical Principles of Psychologists and Code of Conduct and Canadian Code of Ethics for Psychologists.

The Canadian Code of Ethics for Psychologists is based on four principles, including Respect for the Dignity of Persons and Peoples, Responsible Caring, Integrity in Relationships, and Responsibility to Society. The first principle represents the highest priority in professional decision-making and includes the values of "inherent worth, non-discrimination, moral rights, distributive, social and natural justice." The American Ethical Principles of Psychologists and Code of

Conduct includes a reference to general principles of Beneficence and Nonmaleficence, Fidelity and Responsibility, Integrity, Justice, and Respect for People's Rights and Dignity. Within the first principle, professionals are to "safeguard the welfare and rights of those with whom they interact professionally" and "are alert to and guard against personal, financial, social, organizational, or political factors that might lead to misuse of their influence."

Ethical practice requires professional reflection to apply ethical principles in everyday practice. While some efforts have been made to identify minimum professional standards for day-to-day situations, most therapeutic decision-making is not manualized. As well, self-awareness and monitoring are vital to professional self-regulation (Bandura, 1986). In some jurisdictions, ongoing learning integrated via reflective practice is a requirement (Mann et al., 2009).

Cultural Competence

Cultural competence is "the ability to understand, appreciate and interact with people from cultures or belief systems different from one's own" (DeAngelis, 2015). It is a necessity for professional practice and a fundamental competency (Fouad et al., 2009; Sandeen et al., 2018). A great deal of training in this area explores culturally normative behavior with a focus on nondominant or minority groups through the use of didactic methods. However, personal experience, experiential learning, and self-reflection are necessary to develop the awareness and skill (Sandeen et al., 2018; Sue, Arredondo, & McDavis, 1992) to be a competent professional (Epstein, 1999).

Professional Judgment

The complexity of personal and systemic issues encountered in counseling and psychotherapy may not easily fit within existing theories and practice models (Argyris & Schon, 1974; Boud, 1985; Epstein & Hundert, 2002). Judgment "involves critical examination of what is actually going on in situations of practice through a systematic self-reflection, reflective discourse and critically oriented change." In addition to ethical principles and established practices, critical reflection can enhance practice in both common occurrences as well as conditions for which there is no clear precedent (Kim, 1999). Given that our judgment is often heavily influenced by an intuitive sense of emergent patterns

(Dreyfus & Dreyfus, 1986; Johns, 2005), self-awareness improves recognition of the preconceptions that impact on it (Begat, Ellefsen, & Severinsson, 2005; Pack, 2009).

BARRIERS TO REFLECTIVE PRACTICE

Reflective practice requires evaluating what is known while searching for new or better answers. It requires vulnerability and risk taking. It requires self-knowledge of personal values and social and institutional contexts of practice. It often leads to questions about one's practice and degree of fit with clients, agency, and profession. Often, these answers necessitate change. While it is a time consuming and emotionally challenging task for professionals in counseling and psychotherapy, the process is similar to what we expect of our clients (Pack, 2009).

Sharing one's process of RP with a supervisor has potential benefits and drawbacks (Pack, 2009). Such a practice heightens the power differential between the supervisor and supervisee. It exposes the supervisee to additional evaluation and potentially harmful judgment. At its best, however, it invites curiosity, openness, experimentation, tolerance of ambiguity as well as closeness and familiarity (Walker & Rosen, 2004).

Counselors and psychotherapists trained in a positivist tradition of behavioral science (Bennett-Levy, 2003; Lavender, 2003), may find RP to have less potential value in training and therapy practice (Fisher et al., 2015). Evidence-based treatment highlights standardization and decisions based on variables that determine the right intervention for the right client (Stedmon & Dallos, 2009). As such, there may be relatively less emphasis on personal reflection.

Consider a decision you have made in your personal or academic life. It should be significant enough that it stays firmly in memory. But it should also be one that you have already processed and is no longer emotionally charged.

Ask yourself the following questions: (1) what was it? (2) why did I choose it? (3) what happened as a result? (4) if I had the opportunity to consider it again, would I change it? (5) why or why not?

Now, look at your answers to those questions. How long did it take to write answers to 1 through 5? What was it like to answer these questions? What emotions did you experience?

What physical sensations, if any, did you have while reflecting on this? What was relatively easy about this reflection? What was relatively tricky about doing this? What would prevent you from doing an activity like this again? How could you encourage yourself to do another activity like this again?

How Has Reflective Practice Changed?

RP has evolved through paradigm shifts. These shifts are Appropriation, Transformation, Publication, and Conventionalization (Finlayson, 2015). In appropriation, learning focuses on observations of others and transformation is taking knowledge from the observation and altering it so as to be useful to self. In publication, the knowledge is formally recorded and stored, while conventionalization is sharing or showing the knowledge.

Models of Reflective Practice

In *Democracy of Education* (1916) John Dewey writes about the student as more than a passive recipient of knowledge provided by a teacher. Students should learn about their freedom to make decisions and take action in ways that were responsible and ethical. Passivity poses risk for unquestioned acceptance of power structures. His informal reflection models (1933) include the steps of problem identification, observation, hypothesis construction, scrutiny of hypothesis, and finally testing of hypothesis.

David Kolb and Ron Fry add the concept of RP through experiential learning. In their approach, learning comes from experience and is solidified through reflection on that experience. Their four-stage model includes real experience, followed by observation and experience, the formation of concepts, and testing of those concepts in a new situation (1975).

Donald Schön (1983) first uses the term RP. He distinguishes between technical knowledge and the art of practice. Educators, in particular, continue to be influenced by this work. Schön identifies two types of reflective learning, including reflection in action and reflection on action. Reflection in action concerns the reflective process during the event itself and reflection on action concerns the reflection on what happened after the fact.

In 1984 David Kolb adds the component of learning styles to the experiential model. A processing continuum refers to the approach to learning by thinking, and a perception continuum refers to the emotional response to learning. The Kolb and Fry model is modified to include concrete experience (feeling), observation (watching), abstract conceptualization (thinking), and active experimentation (doing). Additionally, ways of processing are included. Diverging occurs with the combination of experience and observation. Assimilating is the combining of conceptualization and observation. Converging is combining conceptualization and experimentation, and accommodating is the combination of experience and experimentation.

Graham Gibbs adds a model of RP in his book *Learning by Doing* (1988). He introduces the ideas of autobiographical self, which is a temporary state of consideration of experiences in order to learn from them. The autobiographical self is private learning insofar as it is embedded in one's learning within a particular sociocultural context. The personal narrative follows the six stages of description, feelings, evaluation, analysis, conclusions, and action plan.

Christopher Johns' (1995) five-stage model of reflective learning is the first conceptualization for professionals. The model is meant to be practiced with a colleague or supervisor and includes attention to both looking in (at one's thoughts and experience) as well as looking out (at the context of the experience). The steps include: description (what was significant?), reflection (what was my purpose?), influencing factors (what influenced my thinking?), could I have dealt with it better? (what other choices did I have?), and learning (how has this changed?) (see Rolfe, Freshwater, & Jasper, 2001).

Stephen Brookfield (1998) offers a view of RP through different lenses on the experience. These lenses include one's personal story leading up to the experience, an account of the experience from the perspective of someone watching to learn about it, the perspective of colleagues, and possible connections to established theory.

CRITICAL REFLECTIVE PRACTICE IN COUNSELING AND PSYCHOTHERAPY

Learning may be described as a set of instructions about what to do, how to do it, and evidence that the steps were followed (Galea, 2012). This approach is culturally based. To illustrate, cultures with a high power differential and uncertainty avoidance (Hofstede, 1980) tend to approach learning this way (Richardson, 2004). It also reflects a structured cognitive approach, in contrast to more esoteric or holistic approaches (Johns, 2005). Critical reflective practice requires the ability to question assumptions (Pollard, 2002). It is also deconstructive and open to change. Without a critical perspective, RP may be only a technical activity that concludes with the views upon which it started (Ixer, 2000). A critical perspective requires that the values of justice and equity enter into the process. In keeping with those values, the knowledges (cultural knowledges, other psychologies, and worldviews) and nonmainstream voices are also necessary (Bleakley, 1999, p. 317). With internal dialogue, where the learner can challenge the accepted values and knowledges, the power to determine which knowledges and values are acceptable and unacceptable becomes an emancipatory experience (Freire & da Veiga Coutinho, 1972; Ixer, 2000).

In a detailed description of RP for counselors and psychotherapists (Sandeen et al., 2018) it is assumed that understanding the concept of culture with distinctions, similarities, and differences between groups is the basis from which culturally based RP occurs. The Reflective Local Practice framework includes knowledge of cultural groups in the region within which one develops or enhances practices through reflection. The biases that emerge from this process are not to be considered problematic, but foundational to the way one perceives, interprets, and makes therapeutic decisions about actions.

The concepts of hot spots, blind spots, and soft spots are areas for continued reflection, personal and professional development. Hot spots are strong emotional reactions based on a personal experience of extreme powerlessness or oppression in one's own life. These are important for practitioners to be aware of. For example, how do they play out in practice? Which compensatory strategies are useful when it occurs (Sandeen et al., 2018)?

Blind spots are points where a lack of self-awareness contribute to unexamined assumptions about another's experience of culture. In contrast to hot spots, these occurrences are rooted in conditions and experiences where the practitioner has held a high degree of social, economic, or political power. Frequently, the experience of power is noted only by those who have relatively less and rarely by those with more. Privilege is essential to recognize. Without an understanding of these blind spots, essential factors are overlooked, or problems may be overidentified (Sandeen et al., 2018).

Soft spots are assumptions that have not been critically examined and permit alterations from established practice. One form of this is lower expectations for individuals with disadvantaged cultural group memberships. Soft spots can arise through over-identification with a client or sympathy for a client (Sandeen et al., 2018).

SUMMARY

- RP benefits therapists and their clients. It is exploring the taken-for-granted aspects of the work. It includes the identification and challenge of therapist assumptions and therapeutic interpretations with a critical lens.
- RP tests what we do not know. It requires answers to questions about what we may be unsure of. It requires vulnerability and includes risk.
- Donald Schön (1983) makes a distinction between technical knowledge and the art of their practice that make excellence possible.
- RP is a progression from a set of techniques to a way of thinking about one's practice.

DISCUSSION QUESTIONS

1. What values underlie your practice? Recall a learning situation in which you were not sure which direction to take. Write a 5-sentence description of the event, including who, what, when, where, and why. In what ways do your values intersect with each of the descriptors? Are there other values in play? Are there other values you hold that did not apply?
2. RP is a critical but constructive activity and way of practice. The critical part is for learning and change. It is still challenging to consider. Think about a recent interaction you have had with a friend or family member where you felt that you handled it very well.

Consider that experience using the questions: What happened? Why did I do what I did? What other courses of action could I have considered? What would have been the likely effects? How do those effects compare to what happened?

3. RP includes not only what the outcome was but how decisions were made. Have a conversation with a peer about the weather and climate change. During the conversation, consider each comment you make and the purpose for each. How did you know what to say and when to say it? Did you hesitate at any point? What was happening in your mind at that time? What does it inform you about your purpose if you did not hesitate?

References

Archer, M. S. (2007). *Making our way through the world: Human reflexivity and social mobility.* Cambridge: Cambridge University Press.

Argyris, C., & Schon, D. A. (1974). *Theory in practice: Increasing professional effectiveness.* San Francisco: Jossey-Bass.

Bagley, C., Abubaker, M., & Sawyerr, A. (2018). Personality, work-life balance, hardiness, and vocation: A typology of nurses and nursing values in a special sample of English hospital nurses. *Administrative Sciences, 8*(4), 79.

Bandura, A. (1986). The explanatory and predictive scope of self-efficacy theory. *Journal of Social and Clinical Psychology, 4*(3), 359–373.

Begat, I., Ellefsen, B., & Severinsson, E. (2005). Nurses' satisfaction with their work environment and the outcomes of clinical nursing supervision on nurses' experiences of well-being—A Norwegian study. *Journal of Nursing Management, 13*(3), 221–230.

Bennett-Levy, J. (2003). Mechanisms of change in cognitive therapy: The case of automatic thought records and behavioural experiments. *Behavioural and Cognitive Psychotherapy, 31*(3), 261–277.

Bleakley, A. (1999). From reflective practice to holistic reflexivity. *Studies in Higher Education, 24*(3), 315–330.

Boud, D. (1985). *Problem-based learning in education for the professions.* Sydney: Higher Education Research and Development Society of Australasia.

Brookfield, S. (1998). Critically reflective practice. *Journal of Continuing Education in the Health Professions, 18*(4), 197–205.

Butani, L., Blankenburg, R., & Long, M. (2013). Stimulating reflective practice among your learners. *Pediatrics, 131*(2), 204–206.

DeAngelis, T. (2015). In search of cultural competence. *Monitor on Psychology, 46*(3), 64.

Dewey, J. (1933). *How we think: A restatement of the relation of reflective thinking to the educative process*. Boston: DC Heath.

Donati, P., & Archer, M. S. (2015). *The relational subject*. Cambridge: Cambridge University Press.

Dreyfus, H. L., & Dreyfus, S. E. (1986). From Socrates to expert systems: The limits of calculative rationality. *Philosophy and technology II* (pp. 111–130). Dordrecht: Springer.

Epstein, R. M. (1999). Mindful practice. *Journal of the American Medical Association, 282*(9), 833–839.

Epstein, R. M., & Hundert, E. M. (2002). Defining and assessing professional competence. *Journal of the American Medical Association, 287*(2), 226–235.

Finlayson, A. (2015). Reflective practice: Has it really changed over time? *Reflective Practice, 16*(6), 717–730.

Fisher, P., Chew, K., & Leow, Y. J. (2015). Clinical psychologists' use of reflection and reflective practice within clinical work. *Reflective Practice, 16*(6), 731–743.

Fook, J. (2002). *Social work: Critical theory and practice*. London: Sage.

Fouad, N. A., Grus, C. L., Hatcher, R. L., Kaslow, N. J., Hutchings, P. S., Madson, M. B., ... Crossman, R. E. (2009). Competency benchmarks: A model for understanding and measuring competence in professional psychology across training levels. *Training and Education in Professional Psychology, 3*(4S), S5.

Freire, P., & da Veiga Coutinho, J. (1972). *Cultural action for freedom* (p. 39). Harmondsworth: Penguin.

Galea, S. (2012). Reflecting reflective practice. *Educational Philosophy and Theory, 44*(3), 245–258.

Gibbs, G. (1988). *Learning by doing: A guide to teaching and learning methods*. Oxford: Further Education Unit, Oxford Polytechnic.

Habermas, J. (1972). *Knowledge and human interests*. London: Heinemann.

Hodgson, D., & Watts, L. (2017). *Key concepts and theory in social work*. London, UK: Macmillan International Higher Education.

Hofstede, G. (1980). Motivation, leadership, and organization: Do American theories apply abroad? *Organizational Dynamics, 9*(1), 42–63.

Ixer, G. (2000). Assumptions about reflective practice. In *Reclaiming social work: The southport papers* (Vol. 1). Birmingham: Venture Press.

Johns, C. (1995). The value of reflective practice for nursing. *Journal of Clinical Nursing, 4*(1), 23–30.

Johns, C. (2005). Balancing the winds. *Reflective Practice, 6*(1), 67–84.

Kim, H. S. (1999). Critical reflective inquiry for knowledge development in nursing practice. *Journal of Advanced Nursing, 29*(5), 1205–1212.

Kolb, D. F., & Fry, R. (1975). Towards an applied theory of experiential learning. In C. L. Copper (Ed.), *Theories of group processes* (pp. 33–58). London, UK: Wiley.

Lavender, T. (2003). Redressing the balance: The place, history and future of reflective practice in clinical training. *Clinical Psychology, 27*(1115), 0022–0167.

Mahalik, J. R., Worthington, R. L., & Crump, S. (1999). Influence of racial/ethnic membership and "therapist culture" on therapists' worldview. *Journal of Multicultural Counseling and Development, 27*(1), 2–17.

Mann, K., Gordon, J., & MacLeod, A. (2009). Reflection and reflective practice in health professions education: A systematic review. *Advances in Health Sciences Education, 14*(4), 595.

Mezirow, J. (1981). A critical theory of adult learning and education. *Adult Education, 32*(1), 3–24.

Napier, L., & Fook, J. (Eds.). (2001). *Breakthroughs in practice: Theorising critical moments in social work.* London: Whiting and Birch.

Pack, M. (2009). Clinical supervision: An interdisciplinary review of literature with implications for reflective practice in social work. *Reflective Practice, 10*(5), 657–668.

Pollard, A. (Ed.). (2002). *Readings for reflective teaching.* London: A&C Black.

Richardson, P. M. (2004). Possible influences of Arabic-Islamic culture on the reflective practices proposed for an education degree at the Higher Colleges of Technology in the United Arab Emirates. *International Journal of Educational Development, 24*(4), 429–436.

Rolfe, G., Freshwater, D., & Jasper, M. (2001). *Critical reflection for nursing and the helping professions: A user's guide.* Basingstoke: Palgrave.

Sandeen, E., Moore, K. M., & Swanda, R. M. (2018). Reflective local practice: A pragmatic framework for improving culturally competent practice in psychology. *Professional Psychology: Research and Practice, 49*(2), 142.

Schön, D. A. (1983). *The reflective practitioner: How professionals think in action.* New York, NY: Routledge.

Stedmon, J., & Dallos, R. (2009). *Reflective practice in psychotherapy and counselling.* Maidenhead, UK: McGraw-Hill Education.

Strupp, H. H. (1980). Humanism and psychotherapy: A personal statement of the therapist's essential values. *Psychotherapy: Theory, Research & Practice, 17*(4), 396.

Sue, D. W., Arredondo, P., & McDavis, R. J. (1992). Multicultural counseling competencies and standards: A call to the profession. *Journal of Multicultural Counseling and Development, 20*(2), 64–88.

Taylor, B. (2004). Technical, practical, and emancipatory reflection for practicing holistically. *Journal of Holistic Nursing, 22*(1), 73–84.

Taylor, E. W. (2017). Transformative learning theory. In *Transformative learning meets Bildung* (pp. 17–29). Rotterdam: Sense Publishers.

Walker, M., & Rosen, W. B. (Eds.). (2004). *How connections heal: Stories from relational-cultural therapy.* New York and London: The Guilford Press.

Watts, L. (2019). Reflective practice, reflexivity, and critical reflection in social work education in Australia. *Australian Social Work, 72*(1), 8–20.

CHAPTER 2

Theories of Learning

A theory is a hunch or prediction. It is also a description and explanation. Scientific theories rely on evidence. Evidence is connected through logic and represented in concepts to explain a phenomenon. Evidence may support, fail to support, or directly contradict a theory.

We rely on formal or informal theories to explain why particular events occur in counseling and psychotherapy. For example, a client does not show up for a scheduled appointment. Why did it happen? What do we do? The answers explain the phenomenon. Consider the following questions:

Is this about the client? (e.g. Is the client avoiding? Did the client forget?)

Is this about the therapist? (e.g. Did I discourage the client? Did I fail to connect with the client? Did I push the client too much?)

Is this about the setting? (e.g. Is this location easily reached? Is the setting comfortable? Is the service affordable?)

Is this about the counseling process? (e.g. Does sitting and talking help this client? Is a quick fix wanted or possible? Will several sessions take too long?)

© The Author(s) 2019
J. D. Brown, *Reflective Practice of Counseling and Psychotherapy in a Diverse Society*, https://doi.org/10.1007/978-3-030-24505-4_2

> How would we know if it was about the client, therapist, setting, or counseling itself? Do we rely on gut instinct? Do we rely on other's professional perceptions (supervisor, colleague)? Do we reach out to the client for their perceptions? What are the facts that matter? How do we choose which evidence matters most and least?

Evidence supports an assertion. The type of evidence required depends on the purpose, context, and application. The findings of high-quality, methodologically appropriate research provide the best evidence. In counseling and psychotherapy, the evidence includes both quantitative and qualitative research findings. Decision-making should combine multiple forms of evidence that balance rigor with expedience (Gold, 2006).

Consider what many would argue is a gold standard for evidence generation in counseling and psychotherapy: randomized-controlled trials. In randomized-controlled trials, an intervention is provided to one of two otherwise identical groups under identical conditions. Differences between groups show that the intervention is the cause of the change. This design has the most scientific weight. However, even the most credible design with rigorous implementation and careful interpretation has limitations.

> Is there sufficient evidence about the intervention with the specific population for the specific issue to supports its use? How much room is there for therapists' differences or deviation from the specific procedures for the therapy to remain effective? How much room is there for clients' differences or deviation from the prototypical client for the therapy to remain effective?

WHAT MAKES EVIDENCE CREDIBLE?

Quantitative research is a deductive process. Constructs develop from theory. Relationships between the constructs either support or fail to support the prediction derived from the theory. A case-control study is a typical design in counseling and psychotherapy research. The method, rigor, and applicability determine its credibility.

Three main questions for a case-control study (Critical Appraisal Skills Programme, 2018):

1. What was the research question and was it answered? How were the participants selected? How did they obtain the data (i.e. were surveys, questionnaires, or observations used?) What were the instruments and procedures? Were they presented with enough detail that another researcher could replicate them?
2. What are the results? How much were the groups different after the intervention?
3. Will the results help? How similar is the population, setting, and risk factors to my setting? Do the results fit in with other results?

Qualitative research is an inductive process. Theory development is one purpose for conducting qualitative research. However, a theory may also be the lens through which questions are asked or results interpreted. While different forms of qualitative studies appear in counseling and psychotherapy literature, a generic approach is shown here. Similar to the case-control example from quantitative research, the method, rigor, and applicability determine the credibility.

Three main questions for a qualitative study (Critical Appraisal Skills Programme, 2018):

1. What was the goal of the study? How were the participants selected? How did they get the data (i.e. were interviews, focus groups, observations, with recordings or notes used?) Has the researcher made their purpose and role in the study clear? How many steps and procedures or processes were described and exemplified in the analysis?
2. What are the results? How precise are the results? Are a range of quotes from participants included?
3. Will the results help? How much can the results be transferred to practice in my setting? (i.e. how similar is the population, setting, and experience). Do the results fit with theory or practice?

RELATIONSHIPS BETWEEN THEORY,
EVIDENCE, AND PRACTICE

Consider your counseling and psychotherapy experience. Where does the information you rely upon most often come from? Is it intuition, theory, or research? Under what circumstances is intuition the best source? When is it least preferred? When is theory the best source? When is it least preferred? When is research the best source? When is it least preferred? What is the most credible type of research evidence to you? Is it qualitative, qualitative, or a mixture of both? What are the circumstances under which qualitative is most or least preferred? Under what circumstances is quantitative most and least preferred?

Theories of Counseling and Psychotherapy

In a theoretical synthesis paper, Western theories of counseling and psychotherapy describe change processes as varying according to three qualities. These qualities include the nature of the individual, the relationship between social and personal functioning, and causality. Three concepts that represent distinctions along these qualities include the autonomous, expressivist, and the social individual. An autonomous individual makes change through the use of cognitive processes, while expressivists the innate desire to self- actualize is the basis for change. From a social perspective, individuals are interdependent, and the mind develops as a result of interactions (Stacey, 2006) (Table 2.1).

Another distinction concerns periods of development. The first force, psychodynamic theories, have been profoundly influential but have limited evidence supporting their effectiveness. Freud's psychodynamic view (Thompson, 2018) assumed that irrational and unconscious forces determine individual behavior. Problems are a result of unconscious content that manifests as defensive patterns of action. The goal of therapy is to promote insight into unconscious forces through rational processing. Freedom of choice exists via insight. Adler's view assumed that early life experiences are profoundly influential. Problems are the product of inferiority and the desire for perfection to cope via task mastery

Table 2.1 Theories compared

	Nature of the individual	Relationship between the individual and context	Nature of causality	Associated theories	
Autonomous	Rational	Independent	Cognitive processes	Psychodynamic Cognitive-behavioral	Social Justice
Expressivist	Self-actualizing	Independent	Holistic processes	Humanistic	
Social	Cultural	Interdependent	Collective processes	Contextual Systemic	

(Sperry, 2018). The goal of therapy is to enhance social responsibility and change self-defeating patterns.

Behavioral and cognitive-behavioral theories in the second force are commonplace in counseling and psychotherapy. They have a well-established research base with a great deal of evidence. Behavioral theory draws from classical and operant conditioning (Russell-Chapin, 2016), in that associations influence all behavior with one's physiology and the consequences of actions. Problems are the result of unhelpful associations and prior results. The goal of therapy is to establish helpful connections between behavior and its consequences. Cognitive-Behavioral Theory (Dobson & Dozois, 2019) focuses on the relationship between thoughts and actions. Problems are rooted in illogical thinking about behavior and outcomes. Goals of therapy are to improve the accuracy of thought from which behavior will become more adaptive. Rational Emotive Behavior Therapy (Ellis, 2019) is about the philosophy held by an individual and how the specific thoughts stemming from it form unrealistic expectations of self and others. Problems are rooted in irrational thinking. The goal of therapy is to aggressively challenge irrational thoughts to the point where the challenging process becomes habitual. Cognitive Therapy (Beck, Davis, & Freeman, 2015) is about the automatic thoughts that are interpretations of what is taking place. Problems are the result of biased or distorted thoughts. The goal of therapy is to become aware of unhelpful thinking patterns and to replace with more adaptive thoughts. Reality Therapy (Wubbolding, 2017) focuses on the need for taking personal responsibility to meet one's needs for belonging, power, freedom, and fun. Problems are the result of failing to take responsibility for one's behavior. The goal of therapy is to recognize thinking that removes self-responsibility and replace it with acceptance of responsibility.

Humanistic theories in the third force have been particularly influential on therapeutic relationship development but have moderate to low supporting research evidence. In existential theory (Van Deurzen & Arnold-Baker, 2018), the focus is on the givens of life such as death, meaninglessness, and anxiety. Problems are the result of failing to recognize and respond to these issues. The goal of therapy is to confront these issues, create meaning and be fully human. In person-centered theory (Bazzano, 2016) the focus is on being the naturally good, trustworthy, realistic, and self-directed person one naturally is to become. Problems are the result of neglecting the positive aspects of self, and the goal of therapy is to experience an empathetic other who can redirect understanding of self into an adaptive and fulfilling view.

The fourth force includes contextual and systemic theories for which there is moderate research evidence. Feminist theories (Brown, 2018) attend to relationships and interconnections between political and personal experience. Problems are the result of unequal power relations on those who are disadvantaged. The goal of therapy is to empower self and make a change that alters the social environment. Family systems theories (Beckvar & Beckvar, 2017) recognize self-in-relation to others and characterize problems as the result of imbalanced, undifferentiated, or inequitable relationships. The goal of therapy is to bring members to a shared understanding and collective responsibility for changing relationships. Constructivist theories (Paz, Pucurull, & Feixas, 2016) present reasonable alternative perspectives on experiences. Problems occur when one's story is problem-focused and when problems become self-defining and limiting. The goals of therapy are to construct new stories focusing on solutions instead of the problems. Multicultural theories (Sue, Sue, Neville, & Smith, 2019) view the individual as a cultural being who is inseparable from history, geography, and customs. Problems occur when perceptions of self and others exist in outdated or inaccurate interpretations of meaning relative to one's cultural perspective. The goals of therapy are to identify, accept, and live in ways consistent with one's cultural values.

Social justice theories are emerging as the fifth force in counseling and psychotherapy. They explicitly attend to sociopolitical forces that produce inequities. Experiences of oppression diminish the potential for and experience of well-being. A social justice approach to counseling "refers to using all of the methods of counselling and psychology to confront injustice and inequality in society" (Kiselica & Robinson, 2001, p. 387). Changes occur as a result of deliberate effort through both intrapersonal and community interventions "to minimize oppression and injustice in favor of equality, accessibility, and optimal developmental opportunities for all members of society" (Kennedy & Arthur, 2014, p. 188). Notably, therapies in this category attend to the use and liberating effects of culturally based psychotherapies as well as the recognition of forces outside of the individual as legitimate targets of intervention (see Table 2.2).

In the following table, highlight the assumptions that resonate for you. They do not need to be within the same school of thought. Once you have identified the assumptions that make the most sense to you consider which schools you most loosely align with. In the section that follows, through the lens of experiential learning, identify the ways that you often rely upon to identify these assumptions.

EXPERIENTIAL LEARNING

Learning may be defined as "a relatively permanent change in behaviour with behaviour, including both observable activity and internal processes such as thinking, attitudes and emotions" (Burns, 1995, p. 99). This definition includes motivation and recognizes that learning may not be immediately apparent. Major theories include sensory stimulation, reinforcement, cognitive-gestalt, holistic, facilitation, and experiential learning theory. In Sensory Stimulation Theory, stimulation of the senses is critical, and the more senses activated, the more influential the learning. In Reinforcement theory, what occurs after a behavior is what determines the likelihood of that behavior happening again with positive consequences being the most powerful. Cognitive-Gestalt approaches place emphasis on experience, meaning, problem-solving, and insights. In Holistic learning theory, the "individual personality consists of many elements... specifically... the intellect, emotions, the body impulse (or

Table 2.2 Theories and assumptions

Schools of thought	Assumptions made					Unit of focus	Processes for change	Ingredients for change	Distance between client and therapist
	Human agency	Source of energy	Human nature	Time orientation					
Psychodynamic	Determined not free	Unconscious forces	Pessimism about human nature	Past oriented		Individual coping with past	Intellectualizing unconscious content	Focus on the interpretation	Power distance is high
Behavioral and Cognitive-Behavioral	Free not determined	Conscious and sensory forces	Optimism about human nature	Present oriented		Individual on measurable change	Intellectual and behavioral training	Focus on rehearsal	Moderate
Humanistic	Free not determined	Holistic (emotional, physical, spiritual, and social) forces	Optimism about human nature	Present oriented		Individual in communion with others	Self-actualization through self-discovery	Focus on meaning	Moderate
Contextual and Systemic	Interdependent	Systemic forces	Optimism about human nature and systems	Past, present and future-oriented		Individuals within systems	Self-in-relation through dialogue	Focus on relationships	Low
Social Justice	Immersed	Structural forces	Optimism about human nature, pessimism about structures	Past, present, and future-oriented		Individuals against structures	Fairness through personal and social action	Focus on social, economic, and political structures	Variable

desire), intuition and imagination" (Laird, 1985, p. 121) which require activation for active learning. Facilitation theory emphasizes the role of an educator who establishes a comfortable setting in which learners take risks and consider new ideas.

In cross-cultural learning, experiential learning theory is highly influential. Kolb's (1984) experiential learning theory is "a holistic process of adaptation to the world" (Kolb, 1984, p. 31). Reflection is fundamental in this model. Experiential learning theory distinguishes between learning abilities, style, skills as well as flexibility and adaptation. As you review these definitions, consider where your learning strengths lie.

Learning Abilities

Experiential learning abilities refer to four stages of concrete experience, observation and reflection, abstract conceptualization, and experimentation. Concrete experience (CE) concerns presence and subjectivity in interpersonal relations. It includes intuitive understanding, sensitivity as well as openness and openness to ambiguity. Abstract conceptualization (AO) focuses on precision, rational processes, logic and systematic planning. Observation and reflection (RO) focus on watching and listening to infer meaning in situations from different perspectives. Active experimentation (AE) is efficient, about taking action, getting things done, and taking chances.

Learning Styles

Learning styles are combinations of preferred learning abilities (Kolb, 1984; Kolb & Fry, 1975). These come from personal preference as well as social, cultural, and environmental factors. A diverging style is based on CE and RO and marked by creativity, imagination, and emotionality. A converging style is based on AC and AE and is characterized by practical problem-solving. An assimilating learning style is based on AC and RO and characterized by logic and abstract understanding. An accommodating learning style is based on CE and AE and characterized practical applications and use of intuition.

Learning Skills

Skills are specific to situations and abilities to be successful on a particular task. Interpersonal skills, helping and empathizing are highlighted in Concrete Experience, while perceptual abilities and gathering information are prominent in Reflection and Observation. Abstract Conceptualization includes technical knowledge and information synthesis, while Active Experimentation centers on setting goals, taking the initiative and direct action (Yamazaki & Kayes, 2004).

THEORY-IN-USE

A view of human learning described by Argyris and Schön (1974) is particularly appropriate to reflective practice in counseling and psychotherapy. The critical contribution of this view is the distinction between espoused theories and theories-in-use. All actions have a map or design. That is, the action is not accidental. It is purposive. We are also responsible for it. These maps are used to take action and they also reflect a theory. That theory is something of which we are often not aware. It is also often different from the theory we espouse. Therefore, two theories are operating at any time. The theory-in-use is the theory upon which our actions are based, and the espoused theory is the theory we tell ourselves and others that we are following. Argyris and Schön propose questions for interrogating espoused theories and theories-in-use. Are the theories internally consistent? Are the theories effective? Is there congruence between espoused theories and theories-in-use?

Improved consistency between these theories will enhance effectiveness (Schofield & Grant, 2013). Reflective practice is a means by which to develop congruence between espoused theories and theories-in-use (O'Hara & Schofield, 2008). It assists by enhancing awareness of the theories by which we take action and in doing so, bring greater awareness into the theories we believe are essential. Through reflective practice, therapists will be increasingly aware of the worldview and values that are believed to underlie actions, and the worldview and values implied by their actions. A more consistent and deliberate as well as helpful practice is the result (Gordon, 2004).

There are three components to theories in use. These include a governing variable, action strategy, and consequences (Greenwood, 1998). The governing variable and action strategy have consequences. Consequences can impact on the action strategy and the governing variable. The governing variable refers to values that matter and are believed to inform our actions. There can be many governing variables operating in any situation. Sometimes, there are conflicts and trade-offs between governing variables. Action strategies are what is done to apply and manage governing variables. Consequences include effects on self and others, as well as the effectiveness of the action strategy itself.

If the consequences occur, the theory-in-use is confirmed. If the consequences do not occur, then one of two possibilities are the case: single or double-loop learning (Kerr, 2010). In single-loop learning, a new action strategy is considered to replace the one employed in order to bring consistency between expectation and outcome. In double-loop learning, the governing principles, as well as the action strategy, are replaced. The difference is that in single loop, the norms are unchallenged, and changes occur within those norms. In double-loop, the norms themselves are challenged and changed. Single-loop learning is best for identifying something a systematic or technical problem and solutions (e.g. doing things right), and double-loop for understanding what the problem is and why it is happening (e.g. doing the right thing).

There is often tension between the norms within which one works and the personal values held by the staff. For example, Savaya and Gardner (2012) examined the beliefs and practices of community agencies' social workers. They found that workers' values of empathy, tolerance, and understanding included partnerships with clients that translated into a client-centered approach. However, actions centered on agency principles and practices translated into an organization-centered approach.

Double-Loop Learning

If double-loop learning is less often utilized but offers more range for action and outcomes, there is a benefit to recognizing and employing it. Theories-in-use have little variability, but espoused theories have a great deal of variability. Most theories in use fall into one of two patterns. In Model 1, the governing variables involved inhibit double-loop learning and in Model 2, the governing variables promote it (Anderson, 1994, 1997).

Governing variables in Model 1 are primarily competitive and defensive. The purpose is to achieve the outcome with an emphasis on rationality and suppression of feelings or discomfort. Primary strategies are to control the environment and protect the self. They manifest as believing that one's assumptions are correct, discouraging inquiry, making covert attributions and judgments, as well as leaving out embarrassing facts

(Anderson, 1994, 1997). Relationships are low in freedom of choice and often defensive. Evidence for Model 1 is in theories of use. They include low honesty, risk, and potential for growth.

Most people espouse Model 2 (Anderson, 1994, 1997). Governing variables in Model 2 concern validity, freedom, and internal commitment. The purpose is to share influence and involvement in then plan and action. Conflicting views are brought to the surface as is the need for continued evaluation for improvement. There is high honesty, freedom of choice, as well as risk and potential for growth (Anderson, 1994, 1997). Validity of information depends on the expression of beliefs, feelings, and intentions. In Model 2, fundamental assumptions are tested, hypotheses are publicly evaluated, procedures can be disconfirmed, and effectiveness determined (Anderson, 1994, 1997).

Consider the following examples of common conventions in counseling and psychotherapy practice. (1) The 50-minute hour. (2) 28-day treatment. (3) Sessions spent sitting in a therapist's office. Why are these conventions? What alternatives are there to these practices? Are there contradicting ideas of what is and what could be? How do we rationalize differences between what is appropriate versus what is done?

CRITICAL CONSCIOUSNESS

Critical consciousness is a means to challenge assumptions of theories on their consistency with personal values. It is "The ability to perceive social, political, and economic contradictions and to take action against the oppressive elements of reality" (Freire 2000, p. 35). It is as much a spiritual, moral, and philosophical process as much as it is intellectual and emotional. Mezirow (2016, p. 13) talks about "being aware of our awareness" of power and privilege. Three concepts associated with social consciousness and change, including critical reflection, critical motivation, and critical action. Critical reflection (Diemer, Rapa, Park, & Perry, 2017; McWhirter, McWhirter, McWhirter, McWhirter, & McWhirter, 2016) focuses on fairness and equity (e.g. critical awareness and analysis about inequities based on political representation, income, and employment differences). Critical motivation is agency (e.g. capable and motivated to make change happen). Finally, critical action is behavior (e.g. responding to unfair interpersonal treatment) and sociopolitical participation (e.g. involvement in social action, groups that promote justice).

Development

There are five stages of critical consciousness, including naiveté, acceptance, naming and resistance, redefinition and reflection, and multi-perspective integration (Freire, 1985). Naiveté is an unawareness of self as a cultural person, one's cultural identity as similar and different from others. Acceptance is a state of early awareness of difference and lack of fairness that may be passive (e.g. accepting that high poverty neighborhoods exist) or active (e.g. participating in an anti-poverty march). Naming and resistance include labeling of the differences between identities and their relative status in society. For Freire, this is the beginning of critical consciousness. Redefinition and reflection are the explicit attention to the sociopolitical hierarchies within which one exists. Multi-perspective integration is where the context and identities interact to produce advantage and disadvantage.

SUMMARY

- Theories describe and explain phenomena. We rely on both informal and established theories to interpret events in counseling and psychotherapy.
- Research may be used to explore theory, enrich theory, create theory or test hypotheses derived from theory. Quantitative research is a deductive process. Qualitative research is an inductive process.
- An essential view of human learning as described by Argyris and Schön is particularly appropriate to reflective practice in counseling and psychotherapy. Two theories are operating at any time. The theory-in-use is the theory upon which our actions are based, and the espoused theory is the theory we tell ourselves and others that we are following.
- Critical consciousness a means to challenge assumptions based on their consistency with critical personal values. It is "The ability to perceive social, political, and economic contradictions and to take action against the oppressive elements of reality" (Freire, 2000, p. 35). It is as much a spiritual, moral, and philosophical process as much as it is intellectual and emotional.

DISCUSSION QUESTIONS

1. Which theories are most influential to the profession? Which are most influential in your work setting? Which are most influential to you, personally? How do these vary? Why would you choose one over another?

2. How do you decide what evidence is most credible? Do you find yourself more drawn to theoretical explanations or research findings or both? Are there circumstances where you give higher priority to one over the other?

3. Intuition, as a source of information and evidence, is not highly valued for its theoretical contributions. However, it often carries weight in personal decision-making. How does your intuition help you determine the best evidence and theoretical explanation?

REFERENCES

Anderson, L. (1994). *Espoused theories and theories-in-use: Bridging the gap (Breaking through defensive routines with organisation development consultants)* (Unpublished Master of Organisational Psychology thesis). University of Queensland.

Anderson, L. (1997). *Argyris and Schon's theory on congruence and learning* [Online]. Available at http://www.aral.com.au/resources/argyris.html.

Argyris, C., & Schön, D. A. (1974). *Theory in practice: Increasing professional effectiveness.* New York: Jossey-Bass.

Bazzano, M. (2016). The conservative turn in person-centered therapy. *Person-Centered & Experiential Psychotherapies, 15*(4), 339–355.

Beck, A. T., Davis, D. D., & Freeman, A. (Eds.). (2015). *Cognitive therapy of personality disorders.* New York: Guilford Publications.

Becvar, R. J., & Becvar, D. S. (2017). *Systems theory and family therapy: A primer.* London: Rowman & Littlefield.

Brown, L. S. (2018). *Feminist therapy.* Washington, DC: American Psychological Association.

Burns, S. (1995). Rapid changes require enhancement of adult learning. *HR Monthly*, pp. 16–17.

Critical Appraisal Skills Programme. (2018). *CASP (Case control study) Checklist* [online]. Available at https://casp-uk.net/wp-content/uploads/2018/01/CASP-Case-Control-Study-Checklist-2018.pdf. Accessed July 6, 2019.

Diemer, M. A., Rapa, L. J., Park, C. J., & Perry, J. C. (2017). Development and validation of the Critical Consciousness Scale. *Youth & Society, 49*(4), 461–483.

Dobson, K. S., & Dozois, D. J. (Eds.). (2019). *Handbook of cognitive-behavioral therapies*. New York: Guilford Publications.

Ellis, A. (2019). Early theories and practices of rational emotive behavior therapy and how they have been augmented and revised during the last three decades. In *Advances in REBT* (pp. 1–21). Cham: Springer.

Freire, P. (1985). *The politics of education: Culture, power, and liberation*. Westport, CT: Greenwood Publishing Group.

Freire, P. (2000). *Pedagogy of the oppressed*. New York: Herder and Herder.

Gold, I. (2006). *What is evidence? A workshop for CIDA policy analysts*. Ottawa: Canadian Health Services Research Foundation.

Gordon, C. (2004). Counsellors' use of reflective space. *Counselling and Psychotheraphy Research, 4*(2), 40–44.

Greenwood, J. (1998). The role of reflection in single and double loop learning. *Journal of Advanced Nursing, 27*(5), 1048–1053.

Mezirow, J. (2016). A critical theory of adult learning and education. *Adult Education, 32*(1), 3–24.

Kennedy, B. A., & Arthur, N. (2014). Social justice and counselling psychology: Recommitment through action. *Canadian Journal of Counselling and Psychotherapy/Revue Canadienne de Counseling et de Psychothérapie, 48*(3), 186–205.

Kerr, P. A. (2010). *Conceptions and practice of information literacy in academic libraries: Espoused theories and theories-in-use* (Doctoral dissertation). Graduate School-New Brunswick, Rutgers University.

Kiselica, M. S., & Robinson, M. (2001). Bringing advocacy counseling to life: The history, issues, and human dramas of social justice work in counseling. *Journal of Counseling & Development, 79*(4), 387–397.

Kolb, D. (1984). *Experiential learning: Experience as the source of learning and development*. Upper Saddle River, NJ: Prentice-Hall.

Kolb, D., & Fry, R. (1975). Towards a theory of applied experiential learning. *Theories of group processes*. Reading, MA: Addison Wesley.

Laird, D. (1985). *Approaches to training and development*. Reading, MA: Addison-Wesley.

McWhirter, J. J., McWhirter, B. T., McWhirter, E. H., McWhirter, A. C., & McWhirter, R. (2016). *At risk youth*. Toronto: Nelson Education.

O'Hara, D., & Schofield, M. J. (2008). Personal approaches to psychotherapy integration. *Counselling and Psychotherapy Research, 8*(1), 53–62.

Paz, C., Pucurull, O., & Feixas, G. (2016). Change in symptoms and personal construct structure in anxiety disorders: A preliminary study on the effects of constructivist therapy. *Journal of Constructivist Psychology, 29*(3), 231–247.

Russell-Chapin, L. A. (2016). Integrating neurocounseling into the counseling profession: An introduction. *Journal of Mental Health Counseling, 38*(2), 93–102.

Savaya, R., & Gardner, F. (2012). Critical reflection to identify gaps between espoused theory and theory-in-use. *Social Work, 57*(2), 145–154.

Schofield, M. J., & Grant, J. (2013). Developing psychotherapists' competence through clinical supervision: Protocol for a qualitative study of supervisory dyads. *BMC Psychiatry, 13*(1), 12.

Sperry, J. (2018). Evidence-based Adlerian therapy. *The Journal of Individual Psychology, 74*(3), 245–246.

Stacey, R. (2006). Theories of change in therapeutic work. *Clinical Child Psychology and Psychiatry, 11*(2), 191–203.

Sue, D. W., Sue, D., Neville, H. A., & Smith, L. (2019). *Counseling the culturally diverse: Theory and practice.* Hoboken, NJ: Wiley.

Thompson, C. (2018). *Psychoanalysis: Evolution and development.* New York: Routledge.

Van Deurzen, E., & Arnold-Baker, C. (2018). *Existential therapy: Distinctive features.* New York: Routledge.

Wubbolding, R. (2017). *Counselling with reality therapy.* New York: Routledge.

Yamazaki, Y., & Kayes, D. C. (2004). An experiential approach to cross-cultural learning: A review and integration of competencies for successful expatriate adaptation. *Academy of Management Learning & Education, 3*(4), 362–379.

CHAPTER 3

Ideologies, Worldviews, and Personalities

Ideology is the ideal way to live. It is the set of ideas about society that create and sustain conditions within which we each may live a good life. Political ideologies reflect the governance structures and functions of an ideal society.

POLITICAL IDEOLOGY

Political ideology is a view of governance rooted in assumptions about human nature and social change. Types of government and leadership vary between as well as within nations and communities. They also produce significant disadvantages and advantages experienced by members of some groups relative to others.

Consider the beliefs about a good society reflected in the orientations to diversity in the terms Cultural Mosaic and Melting Pot. Cultural diversity in the Canadian Cultural Mosaic is the recognition of difference and inclusion of different cultures within the good society. Cultural diversity in the American Melting Pot is the recognition of similarity and blending of different cultures. The Mosaic represents strength in diversity, and the melting pot represents strength through consistency. Each is associated with a different view of public issues and social problems. Neither has produced social, economic, or political equality.

© The Author(s) 2019   33
J. D. Brown, *Reflective Practice of Counseling and Psychotherapy in a Diverse Society*, https://doi.org/10.1007/978-3-030-24505-4_3

PSYCHOLOGY AND IDEOLOGY

Do counseling and psychotherapy serve the dominant political system of their place and time? For example, conversion therapy for sexual orientation is no longer supported. However, the presence of homosexuality in the Diagnostic and Statistical Manual of Mental Disorders until 1987 did reflect prevailing social norms in North America. Prilleltensky (1989) has argued that the discipline and practice of psychology either support the political status quo or challenge it. There are two parts to consider: (1) what is the status quo, and (2) how do counseling and psychotherapy support or challenge it?

A way to think about the status quo is an answer to a question about fairness. Do you believe that life is fair? Do you think your answer would be the same for others in your community, region, nation, or globe? What makes it fair or unfair? Could it be better? Worse? How? Why?

Do you, in your practice of counseling and psychotherapy, seek to change what is unfair? Do those who have been influential to your professional work do so? How? Do any targets for change operate outside of the individual? What is your professional responsibility concerning those targets?

Webster's Third New International Dictionary (1976) defines ideology as "an extremist sociopolitical program constructed wholly or in part on fictitious or hypothetical ideational bases." Ideology has been either ideological delusion or false consciousness (Prilleltensky, 1989). Another view of ideology concerns ideas shared among members of a group to bring them together and bond (Prilleltensky, 1989). A more recent definition refers to "the process of sustaining asymmetrical relations of power–that is, to the process of maintaining domination" (Mayr, 2008, p. 11).

An ideology, then, has several components. First is the belief system itself, including the way of looking at the world with a set of concepts and ideas. Second is the systematic alteration of reality reflected in that belief system. Finally, the belief system either reinforces the status quo or necessitates sociopolitical change (Ryan, 1976, p. 11).

Can counseling and psychotherapy be instruments of social change? Should they be? Are we, as counselors and psychotherapists, to restrict our focus to individuals, families, and small groups? Should we also work with institutions and communities?

Consider the language we use to describe the sources of problems faced by clients. Is it focused on deficits or strengths within the individual? Does that language leave space for responsibility outside of the individual? How are forces not within an individual's control accounted? For example, to secure a job in a community with high unemployment may be defined as a lack of job skills or availability. How should we direct our efforts in such a context?

THE POLITICS OF RESPONSIBILITY

Social policies are government practices concerning resources and their distribution. Four models of policy creation include traditional, rational, incremental, and public choice (Buse, Mays, & Walt, 2012). Traditional approaches are rooted in problem-solving, where the best decision follows an exploration of all possible actions and their expected outcomes to maximize cost to benefit. In a rational approach, a comparison between what is real and ideal provides a continuum along which an acceptable point is chosen. Incremental approaches focus on the consequences of failing to act, and beliefs about what is minimally necessary to avoid those consequences. In public choice theory, economic self-interest and competition between stakeholders determine the action taken.

The word welfare is highly stigmatized. However, the welfare state was constructed to maintain citizenship and participation in the economy (Ebeling, 2007). The welfare state refers to a package of social programs that the government may provide or delegate per public policy. The degree of public investment in welfare and for whom it is accessible varies a great deal.

Three types of welfare states have been described (Castles & Mitchell, 1990). These include social democracy, liberalism, and conservatism. A liberal welfare approach includes only modest benefits to those who fall below a very low minimum standard. The market, in this approach, is the primary means by which to support self and family. A conservative approach is rooted in traditional values, such that support is to be provided by family or private charity and after those sources are exhausted, by government. In a social democratic welfare system, the purpose is to promote equity, by redistribution of resources obtained through taxation that assist those who are the most disadvantaged in the market system.

In contemporary political terms, conservatives favor tradition while liberals favor progress. Ideologies and personalities go together in predictable patterns (Jost, Nosek, & Gosling, 2008; Skitka & Tetlock, 1993). Attitudes about social change and inequality are variables that distinguish between ideological preferences. The left or liberal view and right, or conservative view are consistent with the degree of risk tolerance, uncertainty, and threat. Conservatism is associated with tradition, conformity, order, stability, traditional values, and hierarchy. Liberalism is associated with preferences for progress, rebelliousness, chaos, flexibility, feminism, and social equality (Jost et al., 2008; Skitka & Tetlock, 1993).

Is mainstream psychology conservative? Neutral? Liberal? Why? How do therapists' political views impact on clients who hold similar or different views? How do you feel interacting with a client who holds very different views from your own? How do you handle these differences?

CONNECTING PERSONAL AND POLITICAL

What social issues are most important to you? What are their causes? How do they affect you, your family, and community both positively and negatively? Do they place additional burdens or limits upon members of some groups and not others? How would you know if a client was negatively affected by them?

Consider the following problems that have attracted recent media attention. How do they impact on your practice? What is the potential that they are significant to your clients? How would you know? If they are affecting your client, how would that impact the service you provide?

Hate crime, Poverty, Substance misuse, Unsafe housing, Unemployment

HEALTH DISPARITIES

One way to understand the connections between social issues and personal experiences is through the view of public health. The roots of public health trace back to the recognition of environmental threats to health and a corresponding need to improve conditions to prevent illness. For example, a lack of hygiene—due to inappropriate sanitation practices—is known to cause and transmit disease. Research that led to this conclusion forms a basis for political decision-making about which factors cause which problems and the necessary solutions.

The social determinants of health point to disparities in health and mental health between groups. The World Health Organization (2015), defines social determinants of health as "the conditions in which people are born, grow, work, live and age, and the wider set of forces and systems shaping the conditions of daily life. These forces and systems include economic policies and systems, development agendas, social norms, social policies and political systems." The Centre for Disease Control and Prevention (2015) defines them as "life-enhancing resources" that include food, housing, economic and social relationships, transportation, health care and education (Marmot & Wilkinson, 2005). Social determinants as studied in Canada (Raphael, 2009) include income, education, unemployment and job security, employment and working conditions, early childhood development, food insecurity, housing, social exclusion, social safety network, health services, Aboriginal status, gender, race, and disability.

Do you believe that social determinants affect personal mental health? To what extent do they constrain or facilitate mental health for individual clients? How much change is possible through counseling and psychotherapy with a client who experiences social disadvantage?

There are two main viewpoints concerning differential health status. From a behaviorist perspective, personal decisions determine one's health. Diminished health is due to unhealthy decisions. From a materialist perspective, resource distribution determines health. Diminished health is due to poor living conditions or self-perception relative to advantaged others. Behaviorists locate responsibility in the individual and materialists locate responsibility in the context.

> Which view is closer to your own? What impact does it have on how you see your role as a therapist?

The effects of social determinants on individual mental health occur in different ways. The developmental pathway concerns the transmission of resources that meet basic physical and social needs. The psychobiological pathway concerns the health-damaging stress of unmet needs. The social comparative pathway focuses on limited opportunities and choices that form barriers to healthy behavior. Latent transmission centers on risk exposure at a sensitive time that has an effect later on. Pathway transmission is a risk that places an individual on a specific trajectory. Cumulative transmission is a buildup of risks over time.

> Which view resonates most strongly with you? What impact does it have on how you see your role as a therapist?

WORLDVIEWS

The term worldview comes from the German weltanschauung, which means "a view of the world" (Johnson, Hill, & Cohen, 2011). It is "used to describe one's total outlook on life, society and its institutions" (Wolman, 1973, p. 406). The psychology of worldview first emerged in counseling and psychotherapy by Karl Jaspers, who considered it a suitable framework for viewing the relationship between the individual and others across the lifespan (see Webb, 2009).

Worldviews develop through a process of socialization in the family, community, and society within which one lives. They develop through interactions with caregivers, institutions such as school, and peers (e.g. Berger, 1967; Koltko-Rivera, 2004; Neisser, 2004). The resulting assumptions are shared among group members and evident in behavior, artifacts, and practices (Johnson et al., 2011; Snibbe & Markus, 2005). These views, in turn, filter experience. In the cross-cultural counseling literature, theoretical bases for worldview development have been identified in social learning (Rotter, 1966) and attribution theory (Jones, 1972).

Conceptualization of Worldview

Worldviews in psychology draw upon philosophical and anthropological models for a general structure (Obasi, Flores, & James-Myers, 2009). Two of the most often referenced models may be combined into a single model that includes seven constructs (Johnson et al., 2011). This combined model includes the Cosmology (universe), Ontology (self), Epistemology (knowing and reason), Semiotics (symbols, gestures, and language), Axiology (values and ethics), Teleology (goals and consequences of action), and Praxeology (norms and sanctions). This model is broad and comprehensive. A condensed model focuses on worldview as beliefs about what is and what can be known, what is good, and what one ought to do to reach goals (Koltko-Rivera, 2004).

Spirituality

Spiritual perspectives make important contributions to one's view of the world. While there is a range of spiritual beliefs, organized religion plays a very prominent role. Belief systems change to adapt and reflect the specifics of the social contexts within which they exist. The result is varying systems of beliefs that share the same name. Also, systems of beliefs may merge and blend. In Table 3.1, rough distinctions between some major spiritual belief systems are presented (Adapted from RELIGIONFACTS. com, 2019)

For the descriptions in Table 3.1, consider which most accurately describe your own beliefs as well as which are most distant from your own. What does this tell you about your view of the world? How might it impact upon your practice of counseling and psychotherapy?

Fill in the Spiritual Beliefs Scale by Obasi et al. (2009). In the box beside the item in Table 3.2 check Yes, Somewhat, No for your belief about each.

There are seven factors to this scale. These include Indigenous values, materialistic universe, spiritual immortality, communalism, tangible realm, spiritualism, and knowledge of self. Indigenous values refer

Table 3.1 Spiritual belief systems

	Histories	Practices	Meaning of life	Afterlife	Gods	Scripture
Atheism	Greek philosophy Enlightenment	None	This life is all there is Only humans can help themselves Only humans can help each other	None	No God or Divine Science explains the universe	Marx Freud Feuerbach Voltaire
Buddhism	India Siddharta Gautama (the Buddha) 520 BC	Meditation Mantras Deity worship Mandalas	Avoid suffering Gain enlightenment Release from the cycle of rebirth or Better rebirth by gaining merit	Reincarnation (with no surviving soul) until enlightenment is	Varies Atheistic Polytheistic Buddha taught nothing is permanent	Tripitaka Mahayana Lotus Sutra Others
Christianity	Israel Jesus Christ 30 AD	Prayer, Bible study, baptism, Communion church on Sundays, holidays	All have sinned and are separated from God Salvation is through faith in Christ sacraments Good works	Heaven or hell or purgatory	One God who is a Trinity of Father, Son, and Holy Spirit	The Bible (Old and New Testaments)
Hinduism	India Indigenous religion	Yoga, meditation God or goddess worship pilgrimage Live with purpose/role (dharma)	Humans are in bondage to ignorance and illusion Purpose of gaining release from rebirth, or at least a better rebirth	Reincarnation (with living soul) until gain enlightenment	One Supreme Reality Manifested in many gods and goddesses	The Vedas, Upanishads, Bhagavad Gita, Ramayana Others
Indigenous spiritualities	Rooted in values and beliefs of original inhabitants	Various	Various	Various	Various	Oral teachings and writings
Islam	Saudi Arabia Muhammad 622 AD	Five Pillars: Faith, Prayer, Alms, Pilgrimage, Fasting. Mosque services on Fridays. No alcohol or pork. Holidays related to the pilgrimage and fast of Ramadan	Humans must submit (Islam) to the will of God to gain Paradise after death	Paradise or Hell	One God (Allah in Arabic)	Qur'an (Scripture) Hadith (tradition)

	Histories	Practices	Meaning of life	Afterlife	Gods	Scripture
Judaism	Hebrew Religion 1300 BC	Circumcision at birth, Bar/bat mitzvah at adulthood. Synagogue attendance No pork or other nonkosher foods. Holidays related to historical events	Obey ten commandments Live ethically focus on this life more than the next	Vary No afterlife Shadowy existence heaven	One God, Yahweh (YHVH)	Bible (Tanakh) Talmud
Sikhism	India Guru Nanak 1500 AD	Prayer and meditation Temple (gurdwara), turban Balance work, worship, and charity	Overcome the self Align life with the will of God Become a saint soldier, fighting for good	Reincarnation until resolve karma and merge with God	One God (IkOnkar, Nam)	Adi Granth (Sri Guru Granth Sahib)
Spiritualism	USA, UK, France 1850	Sunday services. Seances and other communication with departed spirits Spirit healing	Body and spirit are separate Morality and contact with spirits affect afterlife	spiritual existence with access to the living depends on the morality of life	Usually based in Christianity	No authoritative texts Learned from advanced departed spirits
Wiccan	Ancient pagan beliefs Gerald Gardner 1900	Prayer, casting a circle, Drawing Down the Moon, reciting spells, dancing, singing, sharing cakes and wine or beer	"If it harms none, do what you will"	Reincarnation until reaching the Summerland	Polytheism Goddesses and Gods Belief in a Supreme Being	No sacred text

Adapted from RELIGIONFACTS.com (2019)

Table 3.2 Spiritual beliefs scale

ϒ	S	N	*Moons, planets, and stars can influence people's moods*
			Some people can cure diseases with words uttered from their mouth
			Children represent a strong connection between the living and the dead
			Spiritually blessed objects can protect a person from harm
			It is possible for some people to learn about the past, or the future, through their dreams
			The nature of reality can be understood through careful meditation
			I feel spiritually connected to my ancestors who have paved the way for me
			Scientific explanations of the universe are superior to spiritual explanations of the universe
			The universe can be reduced to a specific number of independent particles
			Modern science is the best tool for connecting knowledge with reality
			The Big Bang marks the creation of the universe
			Elements of the universe can be purely isolated for scientific analysis
			There is no life after physical death
			Death marks the beginning of a new cycle of life
			My ultimate goal is to improve my community's current condition
			My humanity is partially defined by my contribution to and involvement in a society
			The achievement of my community is more important than my personal achievement
			A person's value should be based on his or her contribution to his or her society
			Only things we can measure should be used to construct reality
			Things that cannot be measured do not exist
			Knowledge is restricted to the limitations of our five senses
			Spiritual and physical health affect each other
			There are visible and invisible dimensions of this universe
			A rock, a river, and my body are compositions of spiritual energy that are derived from the Supreme Being
			The Supreme Being is responsible for the creation of the universe
			Everything in the universe is joined together by spiritual forces
			Spirit is the fundamental connection between all things
			My ultimate purpose is to reach spiritual perfection
			The Supreme Being sent me to this world with a destiny
			It is possible for some people to learn from spiritual entities
			Good and bad, pleasure and pain, and life and death are all two sides of a single reality
			My cultural heritage is often misrepresented and/or ignored in US educational systems
			Learning about my cultural history improves my mental health
			Knowledge of my cultural history is very important to me

Source Adapted from Obasi et al. (2009)

to precolonial (traditional) views about humanity, nature, and knowledge. Materialistic universe refers to physical evidence as truth. Spiritual immortality concerns belief that one lived before birth and will after death. Communalism refers to the sense of responsibility for the welfare of all members of a group or society. Tangible realism refers to the belief in physical reality and information gained through the five senses.

Spiritualism concerns the interconnected and interrelated nature of life created by a Supreme Being. Knowledge of self focuses on knowledge of history, representation in education, and connection to mental wellness (Obasi et al., 2009).

> Which of the items or scales resonate most with you? Why? What might this mean for you when working with a client who does not share that view or experience? What might this mean for a client who does not share your view or experience?

Taxonomic Structure

This structure was developed by Koltko-Rivera (2004) as a means by which to organize significant worldview aspects. In each topic area, consider the lettered topics and circle which of the types in the bulleted list capture your views.

1. Human Nature
   a. Moral Orientation: Good, Evil
   b. Mutability: Changeable, Permanent
   c. Complexity: Complex, Simple
2. Will
   a. Agency: Volition, Determinism
   b. Determining Factors: Biological determinism, Environmental determinism, Intrapsychic, Rational–conscious, Irrational–unconscious
3. Cognition
   a. Knowledge: Authority, Tradition, Senses, Rationality, Science, Intuition, Divination, Revelation, Nullity
   b. Consciousness: Ego primacy, Ego transcendence

4. Behavior
   a. Time Orientation: Past, Present, Future
   b. Activity Direction: Inward, Outward
   c. Activity Satisfaction: Movement, Stasis
   d. Moral Source: Human source, Transcendent source
   e. Moral Standard: Absolute morality, Relative morality
   f. Moral Relevance: Relevant, Irrelevant
   g. Control Location: Action, Personality, Luck, Chance, Fate, Society, Divinity
   h. Control Disposition: Positive, Negative, Neutral
5. Interpersonal
   a. Relation to Authority: Linear, Lateral
   b. Relation to Group: Individualism, Collectivism
   c. Relation to Humanity: Superior, Egalitarian, Inferior
   d. Sexuality: Procreation, Pleasure, Relationship, Sacral
   e. Connection: Dependent, Independent, Interdependent
   f. Interpersonal Justice: Just, Unjust, Random
   g. Sociopolitical Justice: Just, Unjust, Random
   h. Interaction: Competition, Cooperation, Disengagement
   i. Correction: Rehabilitation, Retribution
6. World and Life
   a. Ontology: Spiritualism, Materialism
   b. Cosmos: Random, Planful
   c. Unity: Many, One
   d. Deity: Deism, Theism, Agnosticism, Atheism
   e. Nature-Consciousness: Nature conscious, Nature nonconscious
   f. Humanity–Nature: Subjugation, Harmony, Mastery
   g. World Justice: Just, Unjust, Random
   h. Well-Being: Science–logic source, Transcendent source
   i. Worth of Life: Optimism, Resignation
   j. Purpose of Life: Nihilism, Survival, Pleasure, Belonging, Recognition, Power, Achievement, Self-actualization, Self-transcendence.

Is There Such Thing as a Therapist Worldview?

Five existential themes (Kluckhohn & Strodtbeck, 1961) include those of human nature, social relationships, person to nature, time, and human activity. Human nature is evil, good, or good and evil. Social

Table 3.3 Differences in worldview

Human nature	Evil (−)	Good and evil	Good (*)
Social relationships	Hierarchical	Collateral (+*)	Individual (−*)
Person to nature	Harmony (*)	Subjugation (+)	Mastery (−)
Time	Past	Present (+)	Future (−*)
Activity orientation	Being (+*)	Being-in-becoming (*)	Doing (−)

relationships are hierarchical, collateral, or individual. Person to nature may exist as harmony, subjugation, and mastery. Time orientation is past, present, and future. Activity orientation includes being, being-in-becoming and doing (Mahalik, Worthington, & Crump, 1999).

Research on these themes has found that the constructs differentiate members of different groups. In general, non-majority group (+) members in the United States reportedly found human nature to be both good and evil, nature as suppressive to humanity, time focus on the present, and a being activity orientation (Mahalik et al., 1999). Majority Americans (−) tend to view human nature as evil, relationships as individualistic, mastery over nature, future time orientation, and have a doing activity orientation (Mahalik et al., 1999). Interestingly, differences also exist among therapists (Mahalik et al., 1999; Mau & Pope-Davis, 1993), irrespective of ethnicity or theoretical orientation. Therapists (*) saw human nature as good, relationships as not hierarchical, harmony between people and nature, future-focused orientation, with a being or being-in-becoming activity orientation. See Table 3.3 for a summary.

Cross-Cultural Applications

Worldview is a crucial component in cross-cultural counseling (Ibrahim, 1985), with validated dimensions of experience (Trevifio, 1996). Initial work has converged on the need to recognize within-group differences. Although between-group differences exist, there is considerable diversity within groups. This line of research avoids the potential for stereotyping (Trevifio, 1996).

It is necessary for therapists to identify the salient values and beliefs of an individual client relative to others in their family and community (Carter & Helms, 1987; Myers et al., 1991) so that they may enter the worldview of the client. In a culturally specific view Myers et al. (1991), suggests that attempting to alter a client's worldview can be appropriate if it is in some way associated with the cause or potential solutions to the problem at hand. However, from a culturally relative view, Sue (1978) suggest that the work should always occur within the client's worldview.

> What do you personally view as the preferred approach? How would you feel as a client of a therapist operating from each approach?

Personality Development

> What do you consider to be primary contributors to personality? Why do personalities differ? Consider the nature-nurture issue. Do you see nature or nurture as more influential on individual differences?

Behavioral genetics is one way of studying the environmental and genetic influence on personality. In this approach, a predetermined amount of genetic contribution is assumed based on the degree of a biological relationship. Identical twins share 100% of their genetic material. Twins have the same prenatal environment. If raised in different contexts after their birth, any differences in personality are assumed to be the result of environmental contributions. In the case of adoption, adopted children are more similar to their birth parents than their adoptive parents (Plomin, Loehlin, & DeFries, 1985).

The interaction between genes and the environment begins before birth in the prenatal environment. The process of maturation determines, to some extent, what kind of environmental experiences one is likely to have. For example, if I am a good singer (which, for the record, I am not), I probably had some inclination to practice, and because of the outcomes of that practice, I practiced more and received reinforcement for practicing. In terms of personality not only are the big five approximately 50% genetic, but so are a range of other differences such as cognitive, motivation, values, political beliefs, and self-esteem (Kandler, Zimmermann, & McAdams, 2014).

Interesting questions focus on how genes and environment interact. For example, the effects of genetics decrease over the lifespan, while environmental influence increases (McCrae et al., 2000). In terms of environment, shared environment (i.e. living in the same home) is less influential than non-shared environmental influence (Koeppen-Schomerus, Spinath, & Plomin, 2003).

Personality Traits

> When you think of personality, what comes to mind? What are the specific qualities that you consider?

One way of viewing personality is as a set of traits. These traits include behavior, intellect, and emotion. They change very little over time but differ between individuals. They can be viewed as descriptions of personal qualities. They exist on a continuum. Most people are a combination of both ends with tendencies toward one more than the other.

The Big Five traits include openness, conscientiousness, extraversion, agreeableness, and neuroticism. High openness speaks to the qualities of imaginative and insightful, curious and creative. Low openness is the tendency to prefer the status quo, work with what is concrete and favor consistency. Individuals high in conscientiousness are thoughtful, detail-oriented, and organized. Those low in conscientiousness value freedom and flexibility. Those high in extraversion are social, assertive, talkative, and expressive, while those who are low characterized as reserved, appreciative of solitude, and wanting little attention. High agreeableness traits are trustworthy, altruistic, kind, and cooperative, while low agreeableness traits include competitive, achievement-oriented, and having little concern about others. Individuals high in neuroticism are moody, irritable, and easily upset, while those low in neuroticism are more likely to be consistent, have less worry and stress.

The Big Five Inventory is one measure of these traits and includes the following scales (Soto, John, Gosling, & Potter, 2011). Extraversion includes Sociability (outgoing vs solitary), Assertiveness (leader vs follower), and Energy Level (high activity vs low activity). Agreeableness includes Compassion (soft-hearted vs uncaring), Respectfulness (respects vs rude), and Trust (sees best in others vs finds fault with others). Conscientiousness includes Organization (neat vs unkept), Productiveness (persistent vs procrastination), and Responsibility (dependable vs careless). Negative Emotionality includes Anxiety (worries vs relaxed), Depression (insecure vs secure), and Emotional Volatility (temperamental vs not easily upset). Open-Mindedness includes Aesthetic Sensitivity (likes art/literature vs dislikes art/literature), Intellectual Curiosity (abstract vs concrete), and Creative Imagination (original vs typical).

How do you view yourself regarding the three qualities of each trait? How do you think others see you? Which of these qualities do you appreciate in others? Why? Which of these qualities do you dislike in others? Why?

Implications of Personality Differences

Working alliance in psychotherapy is associated with therapists' personality factors. Trainees rated themselves and were rated by their clients on the working alliance (Chapman, Talbot, Tatman, & Briton, 2009). Those scoring high on neuroticism had higher client ratings of the alliance and lower trainee ratings of the alliance. Those with high openness had lower client ratings of the alliance and higher trainee ratings of the alliance. Those with high agreeableness had lower trainee ratings of the alliance. Average neuroticism and average openness both associated with higher client perceptions of the alliance.

Therapist theoretical orientation is also associated with personality traits (Scandell, Wlazelek, & Scandell, 1997). Those with high agreeableness are more likely hold a cognitive orientation, while those with high openness are more likely to hold humanistic and gestalt orientations. Psychotherapists' personality traits and their therapeutic orientation became more strongly correlated during the later stages of their careers (Topolinski & Hertel, 2007). Regarding the impact of personality traits on the therapist's stress experience in session, those with low extraversion and high neuroticism reported the highest amount of stress (Schumacher et al., 2014).

Political behavior is also associated with personality traits. Individuals participating in Occupy Wall Street activities were administered a personality inventory using the scales of extraversion, agreeableness, conscientiousness, negative emotionality, and open-mindedness. Results found higher emotional stability, extraversion lower agreeableness, and openness with no difference in conscientiousness (Panagopoulos & Lehrfeld, 2015).

How much does personality matter as a therapist? How are personality similarities and differences between clients and their therapists both challenges and assets? What therapist personality are you likely to be most comfortable with? Which are you likely to be least comfortable with? Why?

SUMMARY

- A worldview is what you believe is true (reality), whereas ideology is what you believe is right (morality).
- Worldview is a lens through which oneself and reality are interpreted, including beliefs about what is real, bad, and good, what can be known, pursued, and done.
- Worldviews form through the process of socialization in the family, community, and society within which one lives—interactions with caregivers, institutions such as school, and peers.
- The Big Five personality traits include openness, conscientiousness, extraversion, agreeableness, and neuroticism.

DISCUSSION QUESTIONS

1. What do you imagine a fair society to be? How do the problems that clients bring to therapy interact with the sociopolitical problems of society? Are they in any way related? How? Or Why not?
2. Is there such a thing as a therapist worldview? Which are the most important qualities from your perspective? Does your professional codes of ethics reflect these qualities? Are there any omissions?

3. If there is a substantial genetic influence, what can therapy accomplish? If there is a substantial environmental influence, can therapy counter influences of society, community, and family?

4. Which personality traits are the most desirable for counselors and psychotherapists? Why? Which traits occur often among counselors and psychotherapists? Lowest represented? Why?

REFERENCES

Berger, P. L. (1967). *The social reality of religion*. London: Faber.

Buse, K., Mays, N., & Walt, G. (2012). *Making health policy*. Maidenhead, UK: McGraw-Hill Education.

Carter, R. T., & Helms, J. E. (1987). The relationship of Black value-orientations to racial identity attitudes. *Measurement and Evaluation in Counseling and Development, 19*(4), 185–195.

Castles, F. G., & Mitchell, D. (1990). *Three worlds of welfare capitalism or four?* Graduate Program in Public Policy, Australian National University.

Chapman, B. P., Talbot, N., Tatman, A. W., & Britton, P. C. (2009). Personality traits and theworking alliance in psychotherapy trainees: An organizing role for the five factor model? *Journal of Social and Clinical Psychology, 28*(5), 577–596.

Ebeling, R. M. (2007). Marching to Bismarcks Drummer: The origins of the modern welfare state. *The Freeman: Ideas on Liberty, 57*(10).

Ibrahim, F. A. (1985). Effective cross-cultural counseling and psychotherapy: A framework. *The Counseling Psychologist, 13*(4), 625–638.

Johnson, K. A., Hill, E. D., & Cohen, A. B. (2011). Integrating the study of culture and religion: Toward a psychology of worldview. *Social and Personality Psychology Compass, 5*(3), 137–152.

Jones, E. E. (1972). *Attribution: Perceiving the causes of behavior*. Morristown, NJ: General Learning Press.

Jost, J. T., Nosek, B. A., & Gosling, S. D. (2008). Ideology: Its resurgence in social, personality, and political psychology. *Perspectives on Psychological Science, 3*(2), 126–136.

Kandler, C., Zimmermann, J., & McAdams, D. P. (2014). Core and surface characteristics for the description and theory of personality differences and development. *European Journal of Personality, 28*(3), 231–243.

Kluckhohn, F. R., & Strodtbeck, F. L. (1961). *Variations in value orientations*. New York: Row Peterson and Co.

Koeppen-Schomerus, G., Spinath, F. M., & Plomin, R. (2003). Twins and non-twin siblings: Different estimates of shared environmental influence in early childhood. *Twin Research and Human Genetics, 6*(2), 97–105.

Koltko-Rivera, M. E. (2004). The psychology of worldviews. *Review of General Psychology, 8*(1), 3–58.

Mahalik, J. R., Worthington, R. L., & Crump, S. (1999). Influence of racial/ethnic membership and "therapist culture" on therapists' worldview. *Journal of Multicultural Counseling and Development, 27*(1), 2–17.

Marmot, M., & Wilkinson, R. (Eds.). (2005). *Social determinants of health.* Oxford: Oxford University Press.

Mau, W. C., & Pope-Davis, D. B. (1993). Worldview differences between college students and graduate counseling trainees. *Counseling and Values, 38*(1), 42–50.

Mayr, A. (2008). Language and power: An introduction to institutional discourse. London: A&C Black.

McCrae, R. R., Costa, P. T., Jr., Ostendorf, F., Angleitner, A., Hřebíčková, M., Avia, M. D., … & Saunders, P. R. (2000). Nature over nurture: Temperament, personality, and life span development. *Journal of Personality and Social Psychology, 78*(1), 173.

Myers, L. J., Speight, S. L., Highlen, P. S., Cox, C. I., Reynolds, A. L., Adams, E. M., & Hanley, C. P. (1991). Identity development and worldview: Toward an optimal conceptualization. *Journal of Counseling & Development, 70*(1), 54–63.

Neisser, U. (2004). Memory development: New questions and old. *Developmental Review, 24*(1), 154–158.

Obasi, E. M., Flores, L. Y., & James-Myers, L. (2009). Construction and initial validation of the Worldview Analysis Scale (WAS). *Journal of Black Studies, 39*(6), 937–961.

Panagopoulos, C., & Lehrfeld, J. M. (2015). Big five personality traits and occupy wall street. *Psychology, 6*(15), 1597.

Plomin, R., Loehlin, J. C., & DeFries, J. C. (1985). Genetic and environmental components of "environmental" influences. *Developmental Psychology, 21*(3), 391.

Prilleltensky, I. (1989). Psychology and the status quo. *American Psychologist, 44*(5), 795.

Raphael, D. (Ed.). (2009). *Social determinants of health: Canadian perspectives.* Toronto: Canadian Scholars' Press.

RELIGIONFACTS.com (2019). *World religions.* Retrieved from http://www.religionfacts.com/big-religion-chart.

Rotter, J. B. (1966). Generalized expectancies for internal versus external control of reinforcement. *Psychological Monographs: General and Applied, 80*(1), 1.

Ryan, W. (1976). The art of savage discovery: How to blame the victim. *Blaming the Victim, 226*, 3–29.

Scandell, D. J., Wlazelek, B. G., & Scandell, R. S. (1997). Personality of the therapist and theoretical orientation. *The Irish Journal of Psychology, 18*(4), 413–418.

Skitka, L. J., & Tetlock, P. E. (1993). Providing public assistance: Cognitive and motivational processes underlying liberal and conservative policy preferences. *Journal of Personality and Social Psychology, 65*(6), 1205.

Schumacher, S., Gaudlitz, K., Plag, J., Miller, R., Kirschbaum, C., Fehm, L., ... & Ströhle, A. (2014). Who is stressed? A pilot study of salivary cortisol and alpha-amylase concentrations in agoraphobic patients and their novice therapists undergoing in vivo exposure. *Psychoneuroendocrinology, 49,* 280–289.

Snibbe, A. C., & Markus, H. R. (2005). You can't always get what you want: Educational attainment, agency, and choice. *Journal of Personality and Social Psychology, 88*(4), 703.

Soto, C. J., John, O. P., Gosling, S. D., & Potter, J. (2011). Age differences in personality traits from 10 to 65: Big Five domains and facets in a large cross-sectional sample. *Journal of Personality and Social Psychology, 100*(2), 330.

Sue, D. W. (1978). Eliminating cultural oppression in counseling: Toward a general theory. *Journal of Counseling Psychology, 25*(5), 419.

Topolinski, S., & Hertel, G. (2007). The role of personality in psychotherapists' careers: Relationships between personality traits, therapeutic schools, and job satisfaction. *Psychotherapy Research, 17*(3), 365–375.

Trevifio, J. G. (1996). Worldview and change in cross-cultural counseling. *The Counseling Psychologist, 24*(2), 198–215.

Webb, E. (2009). *Worldview and mind: Religious thought and psychological development.* Columbia: University of Missouri Press.

Wolman, B. B. (1973). *Handbook of general psychology.* Englewood Cliffs, NJ: Prentice-Hall.

CHAPTER 4

Cultural Self 1:
Class, Race, and Ethnicity

Counseling and psychotherapy in a diverse society necessitate awareness of social advantage and disadvantage. Counselors social locations, as viewed by themselves (Kaiser & Prieto, 2018) and by clients (Trott & Reeves, 2018), are increasingly recognized are contributors to effective practice. This chapter focuses on class, race, and ethnicity. In Chapter 5, the focus is on gender and sex, ability, and age. In Chapter 6, the topic of intersectionality discusses how these locations also contribute to a sense of personal identity.

CLASS

When you think of class, what comes to mind? What are the specific aspects that you consider?

Do you see class difference as a social issue? Political issue? Family issue? Personal problem? How so?

Which classes are most and least often represented by therapists in your own experience, as well as by those you have known and worked with? What are the class compositions of their client bases?

© The Author(s) 2019
J. D. Brown, *Reflective Practice of Counseling and Psychotherapy in a Diverse Society*, https://doi.org/10.1007/978-3-030-24505-4_4

How much does class matter as a therapist? How is therapist similarity or difference to the client an asset or hindrance? How could differences between clients and therapists be bridged?

Definition of Class

Social class encompasses both socioeconomic status and subjective social status (American Psychological Association, 2019a). *Socioeconomic status is the social standing or class of an individual or group. It is a combination of education, income, and occupation. Examinations of socioeconomic status often reveal inequities in access to resources, plus issues related to privilege, power, and control* (American Psychological Association, 2019b). Subjective social status is *an individual's perception of his position in the social hierarchy* (Jackman & Jackman, 1973).

Expressions of Class

Class is a form of inequality that is as much about economics as moral standing. Economic resources include income, education, and wealth (Fisher, O'Donnell, & Oyserman, 2017). These are evidenced by possessions and activities (Rucker & Galinsky, 2012). Standing includes status associated with occupation and authority. It is often associated with the type of language used and how one dresses (Moya & Fiske, 2017).

Class is also associated with judgments about moral behavior and lifestyle (Lawler, 2005). Higher class location is perceived to associate with advanced moral standing and the right kinds of standards. It is perceived to relate to evaluations of another's trustworthiness, values and behavior, achievements, and code of conduct (Fiske, Moya, Russell, & Bearns, 2012). Class-based lifestyle differences may be evident in hobbies and interests, tastes, and travel.

Most people in North America perceive themselves to be a member of the middle class. This subjective rating contrasts with the more objective differences between economic standing. About half of the middle class accurately perceive their standing, about two-thirds of the upper middle class undervalue their standing, and about one-third of the working class overvalue their standing relative to others (Sosnad, Brady, & Frenk, 2013). Importantly, these perceptions also extend to the classes of individuals with which one is willing or not willing to associate

(Cohen, Shin, Liu, Ondish, & Kraus, 2017). Those who identify as middle class view most others as middle class, and associate with others perceived to be of the same class.

Self-Location in Relation to Class

> Where do you see yourself in terms of class? Economic indicators are financially based and associated with income, occupation, and possessions. Cultural indicators are socially based and associated with language, lifestyle, and social networks.

Class identity is evident in labels such as high and upper middle class, middle, and lower class, in addition to working class, working poor, and poor. These labels can blend and intersect, such as in the case of the working poor. The meanings carry prestige or stigma. They connote different environments of living and working. The environments have an impact on lifestyle which is associated with interests and activities (Piff & Moskowitz, 2018).

Theoretically, the highest class offers the most opportunities, choice, and lowest exposure to threats from the environment. Middle and upper classes may offer choices and opportunities that allow greater financial independence. Theoretically, the lowest class offers few opportunities, a severely constrained set of choices from which to act, higher exposure to environmental threats, and inadequate resources to address the threats. Research into ways of thinking from a mindset of scarcity (Mullainathan & Shafir, 2013), reflect a tendency to focus on immediate needs instead of longer-term issues, and attention to the most salient matters relative to others that are co-occurring and in urgent need of response. Severe scarcity reduces cognitive performance (Moya & Fiske, 2017).

Attitudinal and Social Barriers

Research on the psychology of class has centered on several themes. These topics impact on the therapeutic alliance. Consider your own beliefs about these topics and their relevance to your sense of self as well as how a client may perceive you. These topics include merit, stigma, and political values.

In each section, consider which of these barriers have you encountered? How can these inaccurate and negatively biased judgments be recognized and addressed in therapy?

Merit is the belief that reward follows from effort and character (Major & O'Brien, 2005). The more productive one is, the more status is possessed. Individuals from a high class tend to favor decisions based on merit, feel that personal effort is all that separates low from high achievement, and believe that the current economy and political environments are fair (Kraus & Tan, 2015). Those with the highest status are happier when they believe status is based on merit (Napier & Jost, 2008), that resources are distributed on the basis of merit (Brown-Iannuzzi, Lundberg, Kay, & Payne, 2015), and that merit is the fairest means of distribution (Kraus & Keltner, 2013).

Stereotypes and prejudice may include judgments of "lazy" and "immoral" (Cozzarelli, Wilkinson, & Tagler, 2001; Lott & Saxon, 2002). Also, individuals may be perceived by those of relatively higher standing to have lower achievement (Batruch, Autin, & Butera, 2017) and competence than themselves (Durante, Tablante, & Fiske, 2017; Moya & Fiske, 2017). Judgments about individuals who are perceived to be from a lower class may include limited initiative and will, planning, and willpower (Fisher 2011).

Another belief held by some is that "the system works if you work it." For example, if one is not climbing the social ladder, it is because they do not want it enough, take enough initiative, or responsibility (Rodriguez-Bailon et al., 2017). The Protestant work ethic takes this a step further by placing God's favor on those who are economically privileged and not on those who are disadvantaged (Fisher 2011). Therefore, may be it is assumed that a great deal of natural motivation exists to work hard, make money, and be financially successful (Fisher 2011; Sainz, Martínez, Sutton, Rodríguez-Bailón, & Moya, 2019).

Do you agree with the sentiments expressed in these paragraphs? Do they represent beliefs that can be problematic? Why or why not? Do they stereotype, stigmatize, or diminish people? Should such attitudes be challenged by professionals? Should they be challenged in therapy? Under what conditions?

RACE AND ETHNICITY

When you think of race, what comes to mind? How is race different from ethnicity? What do you think of when you think of ethnicity? What are the specific aspects of race and ethnicity that you consider?

Do you see race-relations as a social issue? Political issue? Family issue? Personal problem? How? Do you view interethnic relations as a social issue? Political issue? Family issue? Personal problem? How?

Which races and ethnicities are most and least often represented by therapists in your own experience, as well as by those you have known and worked with? What are the racial and ethnic compositions of their client bases?

How much do race and ethnicity matter as a therapist? How is therapist similarity or difference to the client an asset or hindrance? How could differences between clients and therapists be bridged?

Definitions of Race and Ethnicity

Race typically refers to *shared physical characteristics, such as skin color and facial features* (Verkuyten, 2018). Ethnicity typically refers to *the sameness of a band or nation of people who share common customs, traditions, historical experiences, and in some instances, geographical residence* (Trimble & Dickson, 2005).

Expressions of Race and Ethnicity

In Canada the term "visible minority" is used in legislation. The history of its use begins with the advocacy efforts of Kay Livingstone who organized a national conference for racialized women in 1975. In a subsequent report from the Royal Commission on Equality and Employment its purpose was "to combine all non-whites together as visible minorities for the purpose of devising systems to improve their equitable participation, without making distinctions to assist those groups in particular need." However, in actuality it served to "deflect attention from where the problems are greatest." The cost of creating "visible minorities" in Canada to improve workforce participation grouped those with the lowest and highest participation. Currently, in Canada's Employment Equity Act (1986), visible minorities are "persons, other than Aboriginal peoples, who are non-Caucasian in race or non-white in colour" (Grant & Balkissoon, 2019).

The use of physical characteristics to identify as a visible minority *serves as a proxy for non-White physical appearance, as the word visible and references to non-White color imply* (Roth, 2017).

Is the term visible minority outdated? What is a more appropriate term?

What are the risks and benefits of using a single term to refer to people of color other than Indigenous peoples?

In the United States, racial categories included in the census questionnaire generally "reflect a social definition of race recognized in this country and not an attempt to define race biologically, anthropologically, or genetically" (U.S. Census Bureau, 2019). Categories include White (origins with original peoples of Europe, Middle East or North Africa), Black or African American (origins in any Black racial group of Africa), American Indian or Alaska Native (origins in any original peoples of the Americas), Asian (origins in original peoples of East, Southeast Asia, or the Indian subcontinent), and Native Hawaiian or Other Pacific Islander (origins in original people of Hawaii or Pacific Islands).

Are these five racial categories sufficiently inclusive and exclusive? What purposes do these categories serve? How should these terms be changed?

In the psychological literature, ethnicity has been represented in many ways and with different points of emphasis. These include shared culture, descent, territory, language, history, symbols, mutual recognition, religion, and economic ties (Cartrite, 2003; Zagefka, 2009). Ethnicity may also be understood as affiliation and includes the cultural groups that one chooses to belong to or is seen by others to be a member. Such connections include physical qualities or geographic origins as well as include symbols such as holidays and clothing (Trimble & Dickson, 2005).

Individuals also may claim mixed ethnicity, which is a combination of two or more ethnicities (Batchelder & Root, 1994). Reasons that multiethnic individuals may identify in this way include the security that comes from understanding parts of their heritage, the influence of grandparents on grandchildren to choose, gender alignment between parents and children may affect ethnic socialization, and finally, racism and prejudice against a group makes affiliation important for self-protection and self-confidence (Trimble & Dickson, 2005).

Self-Location in Relation to Race and Ethnicity

All people, regardless of their race, ascribe different psychological meanings to their race. It is this meaning that determines how an individual makes sense of the world and themselves as racial beings (Helms, 1990; Carter & Johnson, 2019).

Do you identify yourself according to race? What descriptors do you use? What does it mean to you to identify yourself in this way?

Scholarly definitions for racial identity, observed race, racial self-classification, reflected race and racial ancestry are used in the literature (Campbell, Bratter, & Roth, 2016; Campbell & Troyer, 2007; Saperstein, 2012). These refer to how we identify, how we believe others see us, how others objectively see us, how we identify when given limited options, how we express our race, and where we locate ourselves historically and geographically. Racial identity includes thoughts, feelings, and behaviors (Carter & Johnson, 2019). Look at each statement in the box below and reflect on what comes to mind.

I identify myself racially as _____.
I think others see me racially as _____.
I identify as ___ when given limited options (i.e. the official defini-
tions in Canada and the United States).
I express myself racially by _____.
I locate myself historically and geographically by _____.

It is the belief of *a common origin that distinguishes ethnic identity from other social identities* (Verkuyten, 2018)...*physical similarities, cultural features, language, religion, and historical events and myths can all play a role in the definition and justification of a common origin* (Verkuyten, 2018). Phinney, Madden, and Santos (1998) *defined ethnic identity as the psychological relationship, attitudes, and emotional salience people attach to their ethnic group* (Bonifacio, Gushue, & Mejia-Smith, 2018).

How do you identify yourself according to ethnicity? What qualities are central to your sense of self as an ethnic person? (e.g. What
languages do you speak? How would you describe your religious
beliefs? What holidays do you celebrate?)

There is a great deal of evidence that genetic differences are more significant within ethnic groups than between them (Bonham, Warshauer-Baker, & Collins, 2005; Smedley & Smedley, 2005). Thus, "construction and choice, rather than blood and inheritance, is now the standard storyline about identity" (Laitin, 1998, p. 12; Sternberg, Grigorenko, & Kidd, 2005; Zagefka, 2009).

Different approaches to racial and ethnic identity include multidimensional, developmental, and patterned. The Multidimensional approach of Sellers, Smith, Shelton, Rowley, and Chavous (1998) emphasizes identity in the context of intergroup relations. Developmental models such as Helms' People of Color Identity Development model (1995) and Phinney's Ethnic Identity Development model (1990) emphasize personal progress over time. Renn's (2008) Identity Patterns approach focuses on personalized combinations of existing or traditional racial or ethnic groups with which one identifies.

In a Multidimensional approach (Sellers et al., 1998) salience, centrality, regarding, and ideology reflect the nature and extent of personal connection with racial identity and values about diversity. Racial salience refers to the degree to which racial identity is essential to self-concept at a time and place. Racial centrality is the degree to which racial identity is important to self-image. Racial regard is one's regard for their race, both public (e.g. how others view people of my racial identity) and private (e.g. how I feel about my own racial identity). Racial ideology refers to how people of the same race should act, including nationalist (i.e. us and them, we cannot live in harmony because of differences), oppressed minority (i.e. same forces that oppress my group have oppressed other groups as well), assimilation (i.e. degree to which working with the system to achieve economic and political goals is desirable/possible), and humanist (i.e. people of my own racial identity have much in common with members of the dominant race).

Developmental models emphasize change over time and maturation to higher levels of awareness and self- definition. For example, People of Color identity development (Helms, 1995) includes conformity (i.e. align with White society), dissonance (i.e. anxiety suppressed because of tension between White and people of belonging), and immersion/ emersion (i.e. favor own group and reject White). Subsequent stages of development include internalization (i.e. becoming flexible in the determination of Whiteness and be more objective in dealings) and integrative awareness (i.e. value of one's oppressed group and connections with other oppressed groups). In this model, progression is reflected by the abandonment of White culture as it related to self-definition, and acceptance of identity as a member of the non-majority group (Carter & Johnson, 2019).

Phinney's (1990) model of identity development includes the three stages of unexamined, search, and achievement. Initially, ethnicity may not be recognized or might be denied in favor of the dominant culture's values and traditions. For some individuals, this is the stage at which their ethnic identity remains. Often what promotes consideration and exploration is an incident or increasing awareness of differences and outward search for information from friends and family, courses and books, as well as travel and life experience. This second stage can also last for a considerable length of time and be a final stage of development. Ethnic identity achievement is what occurs when conscious acceptance of ethnicity and its positioning, with positive attitudes about one's ethnicity and legitimacy of others' ethnicity.

Descriptive models of identity emphasize factors and orientations that contribute to a sense of self. For example, Identity Patterns (Renn, 2008) includes studies with biracial and multiracial postsecondary students in the United States. Different profiles include mono-racial, multiple mono-racial, multiracial, extra-racial, and situational. Mono-racial identity is a choice of one background with which to identify. Multiple mono-racial identities refer to different identifications depending on what one is doing and with whom. Multiracial identity is a blend of ethnic compositions into something new. Extra-racial identity is a rejection of the racial identity idea because of its social construction and origins in dominant, European history. Situational identity is a sense of identity that is more fluid with different aspects, more or less salient in different contexts.

Where do you see yourself concerning these models?
In what contexts are you most aware of your racial or ethnic identity?

Generally speaking, how important to your sense of self is your racial or ethnic identity? How aware are you of others' reactions to people of your race or ethnicity?

How similar and different is your racial or ethnic identity from the identities of the majority of the population where you live? What similarities and differences do you notice between your racial or ethnic identity and others in your community?

Attitudinal and Social Barriers

Sue (2010) distinguishes between modern and aversive racism. Modern racism refers to right-wing conservatives who talk about traditional values or family values. Aversive racism is what liberals practice when they are conflicted between values of equality but harbor negative feelings. Aversive racism is not conscious. It is difficult to identify yet very harmful. It is also not apparent to those holding the beliefs. One way that aversive racism manifests is through microaggressions. Indeed, the personal, structural and relational are all interconnected "Inasmuch as a person who is constantly exposed to hearing language which stigmatizes him/her is distressed by that experience, this is as real a form of oppression as structural discrimination" (Hopton, 1997).

As defined by Sue (2010) "Microaggressions are the everyday verbal, nonverbal, and environmental slights, snubs, or insults, whether intentional or unintentional, which communicate hostile, derogatory, or negative messages to target persons based solely upon their marginalized group membership. In many cases, these hidden messages may invalidate the group identity or experiential reality of target persons, demean them on a personal or group level, communicate they are lesser human beings, suggest they do not belong with the majority group, threaten and intimidate, or relegate them to inferior status and treatment." Three forms of microaggressions include (Sue, 2010): micro-assault, microinsult, and microinvalidation. Micro- assault is explicit denigration that is deliberate and conscious, held and expressed when the person feels safe to do so or just overwhelmed. Microinsult is subtler and not recognized by the person doing it but appearing to the other, such as talking over someone or diverting one's attention when they speak. Microinvalidation is communication that invalidates another's experience.

Have you experienced or witnessed microaggressions? What examples stand out for you? What would make you comfortable enough to tell your therapist about them? What might you do if the one who committed the microaggression was a therapist?

Power differences based on racial identity status have led to the development of a typology that organizes different forms of the therapeutic relationship (Helms, 1984, 1995). The emphasis is not the racial identities per se, but how the statuses combine and interact. There are four different types, including parallel, crossed, progressive, and regressive. A parallel dyad puts the client and therapist at a similar stage of development. In a crossed relationship, the therapist and client hold opposite attitudes about racial groups (e.g. Black therapist, White client, the therapist has anti-White views, and the client has anti-Black views). A progressive relationship is evident by a therapist who has a highly developed racial identity relative to the client. The therapist is therefore sensitive to issues and may be able to connect from a place of having experienced some changes upon which the client is embarking. A regressive relationship is evident when a therapist has less development of their racial identity than the client and is particularly problematic when issues of race come up in the session.

What might you look for in a client to indicate where they are in terms of racial or ethnic identity? What might you look for in a therapist concerning racial or ethnic identity? How comfortable are you, as a client and therapist, discussing issues of race or ethnicity with someone who shares versus does not share your racial or ethnic identity? What might make you more comfortable as a therapist? What might make you more comfortable as a client?

Summary

- Class refers to standing and resources. Role and possessions may reflect it. It is also a judgment of status relative to others.
- Definitions of race refer to physical characteristics. In contrast, ethnicity is a social construction and choice but also a matter of lineage.
- Definitions for racial identity, observed race, racial self-classification, reflected race and racial ancestry refer to how people identify themselves, how they believe others see them, as well as how others objectively see them, as well as how one identifies when given limited options.

Discussion Questions

1. How do social locations, in general, affect counseling and psychotherapy practice? The profession? Therapists and clients? The therapy itself?
2. What do you notice when working with someone who has a very different experience of class than you? What are the signals

that you recognize that differentiate ones class experience from another's?

3. Do you think it is essential to match therapists with clients who share racial and ethnic identifications? Why or why not?

References

Allwood, C. M. (2011). On the foundation of the indigenous psychologies. *Social Epistemology, 25*(1), 3–14.

American Psychological Association. (2019a). *Social class.* Retrieved from https://www.apa.org/pi/ses/resources/class/definitions.

American Psychological Association. (2019b). *Socioeconomic status.* Retrieved from https://www.apa.org/topics/socioeconomic-status/.

Batchelder, T. H., & Root, S. (1994). Effects of an undergraduate program to integrate academic learning and service: Cognitive, prosocial cognitive, and identity outcomes. *Journal of Adolescence, 17*(4), 341–355.

Batruch, A., Autin, F., & Butera, F. (2017). Re-establishing the social-class order: Restorative reactions against high-achieving, low-SES pupils. *Journal of Social Issues, 73*(1), 42–60.

Bonham, V. L., Warshauer-Baker, E., & Collins, F. S. (2005). Race and ethnicity in the genome era: The complexity of the constructs. *American Psychologist, 60*(1), 9.

Bonifacio, L., Gushue, G. V., & Mejia-Smith, B. X. (2018). Microaggressions and ethnic identity in the career development of Latina college students. *The Counseling Psychologist, 46*(4), 505–529.

Brown-Iannuzzi, J. L., Lundberg, K. B., Kay, A. C., & Payne, B. K. (2015). Subjective status shapes political preferences. *Psychological Science, 26*(1), 15–26.

Campbell, M. E., & Troyer, L. (2007). The implications of racial misclassification by observers. *American Sociological Review, 72*(5), 750–765.

Campbell, M. E., Bratter, J. L., & Roth, W. D. (2016). Measuring the diverging components of race: An introduction. *American Behavioral Scientist, 60,* 381–389.

Carter, R. T., & Johnson, V. E. (2019). Racial identity statuses: Applications to practice. *Practice Innovations, 4*(1), 42.

Cartrite, B. (2003). *Reclaiming their shadow: Ethnopolitical mobilization in consolidated democracies* (Doctoral diss.). University of Colorado.

Cohen, D., Shin, F., Liu, X., Ondish, P., & Kraus, M. W. (2017). Defining social class across time and between groups. *Personality and Social Psychology Bulletin, 43*(11), 1530–1545.

Cozzarelli, C., Wilkinson, A. V., & Tagler, M. J. (2001). Attitudes toward the poor and attributions for poverty. *Journal of Social Issues, 57*(2), 207–227.

Durante, F., Tablante, C. B., & Fiske, S. T. (2017). Poor but warm, rich but cold (and competent): Social classes in the stereotype content model. *Journal of Social Issues, 73*(1), 138–157.

Fisher, P. (2011). Performativity, well-being, social class and citizenship in English schools. *Educational Studies, 37*(1), 49–58.

Fisher, O., O'Donnell, S. C., & Oyserman, D. (2017). Social class and identity-based motivation. *Current Opinion in Psychology, 18*, 61–66.

Fiske, S. T., Moya, M., Russell, A. M., & Bearns, C. (2012). The secret handshake: Trust in cross-class encounters. In S. T. Fiske & H. R. Markus (Eds.), *Facing social class: Social psychology of social class*. New York: Russell Sage Foundation.

Grant, T., & Balkissoon, D. (2019). *'Visible minority': Is it time for Canada to scrap the term?* https://www.theglobeandmail.com/canada/article-visible-minority-term-statscan/.

Helms, J. E. (1984). Toward a theoretical explanation of the effects of race on counseling a Black and White Model. *The Counseling Psychologist, 12*(4), 153–165.

Helms, J. E. (Ed.). (1990). *Black and White racial identity: Theory, research, and practice* (Contributions in Afro-American and African studies, No. 129). New York, NY: Greenwood Press.

Helms, J. E. (1995). An update of Helm's White and people of color racial identity models. In J. G. Ponterotto, J. M. Casas, L. A. Suzuki, & C. M. Alexander (Eds.), *Handbook of multicultural counseling* (pp. 181–198). Thousand Oaks, CA: Sage.

Hopton, J. (1997). Towards a critical theory of mental health nursing. *Journal of Advanced Nursing, 25*(3), 492–500.

Jackman, M. R., & Jackman, R. W. (1973). An interpretation of the relation between objective and subjective social status. *American Sociological Association, 38*(5), 569–582.

Kaiser, D. J., & Prieto, L. R. (2018). Trainee estimates of working alliance with upper-and working-class clients. *Counselling and Psychotherapy Research, 18*(2), 154–165.

Kraus, M. W., & Keltner, D. (2013). Social class rank, essentialism, and punitive judgment. *Journal of Personality and Social Psychology, 105*(2), 247.

Kraus, M. W., & Tan, J. J. (2015). Americans overestimate social class mobility. *Journal of Experimental Social Psychology, 58*, 101–111.

Laitin, D. D. (1998). *Identity in formation: The Russian-speaking populations in the near abroad*. Ithaca, NY: Cornell University Press.

Lawler, S. (2005). Introduction: class, culture and identity. *Sociology, 39*(5), 797–806.

Lott, B., & Saxon, S. (2002). The influence of ethnicity, social class, and context on judgments about US women. *The Journal of Social Psychology, 142*(4), 481–499.

Major, B., & O'brien, L. T. (2005). The social psychology of stigma. *Annual Review of Psychology, 56,* 393–421.

Moya, M., & Fiske, S. T. (2017). The social psychology of the Great Recession and social class divides. *Journal of Social Issues, 73*(1), 8–22.

Mullainathan, S., & Shafir, E. (2013). *Scarcity: Why having too little means so much.* Picador: Macmillan.

Napier, J. L., & Jost, J. T. (2008). Why are conservatives happier than liberals? *Psychological Science, 19*(6), 565–572.

Phinney, J. S. (1990). Ethnic identity in adolescents and adults: A review of research. *Psychological Bulletin, 108,* 499–514.

Phinney, J. S., Madden, T., & Santos, L. J. (1998). Psychological variables as predictors of perceived ethnic discrimination among minority and immigrant adolescents. *Journal of Applied Social Psychology, 28*(11), 937–953.

Piff, P. K., & Moskowitz, J. P. (2018). Wealth, poverty, and happiness: Social class is differentially associated with positive emotions. *Emotion, 18*(6), 902.

Renn, K. A. (2008). Research on biracial and multiracial identity development: Overview and synthesis. *New Directions for Student Services, 2008*(123), 13–21.

Rodriguez-Bailon, R., Bratanova, B., Willis, G. B., Lopez-Rodriguez, L., Sturrock, A., & Loughnan, S. (2017). Social class and ideologies of inequality: How they uphold unequal societies. *Journal of Social Issues, 73*(1), 99–116.

Roth, W. D. (2017). Methodological pitfalls of measuring race: International comparisons and repurposing of statistical categories. *Ethnic and Racial Studies, 40*(13), 2347–2353.

Rucker, D. D., & Galinsky, A. (2012). Compensatory consumption. In A. A. Ruvio & R. W. Belk (Eds.), *The Routledge companion to identity and consumption* (pp. 207–215). Abingdon, OX: Routledge/Taylor & Francis Group.

Sainz, M., Martínez, R., Sutton, R. M., Rodríguez-Bailón, R., & Moya, M. (2019). *Less human, more to blame: Animalizing poor people increases blame and decreases support for wealth redistribution.* Group Processes & Intergroup Relations. https://doi.org/10.1177/1368430219841135.

Saperstein, A. (2012). Capturing complexity in the United States: Which aspects of race matter and when? *Ethnic and Racial Studies, 35*(8), 1484–1502.

Sellers, R. M., Smith, M. A., Shelton, J. N., Rowley, S. A., & Chavous, T. M. (1998). Multidimensional model of racial identity: A reconceptualization of African American racial identity. *Personality and Social Psychology Review, 2*(1), 18–39.

Smedley, A., & Smedley, B. D. (2005). Race as biology is fiction, racism as a social problem is real: Anthropological and historical perspectives on the social construction of race. *American Psychologist, 60*(1), 16.

Sosnad, B., Brady, D., & Frenk, S. (2013). Class in name only: Subjective class identity, objective class position, and vote choice in American Presidential elections. *Social Problems, 60,* 81–99.

Sternberg, R. J., Grigorenko, E. L., & Kidd, K. K. (2005). Intelligence, race, and genetics. *American Psychologist, 60*(1), 46.

Sue, D. W. (2010). Microaggressions, marginality, and oppression: An introduction. In D. W. Sue (Ed.), *Microaggressions and marginality: Manifestations, dynamics, and impact* (pp. 3–22). Hoboken, NJ: Wiley.

Trimble, J. E., & Dickson, R. (2005). Ethnic identity. *Encyclopedia of Applied Developmental Science, 1,* 415–420.

Trott, A., & Reeves, A. (2018). Social class and the therapeutic relationship: The perspective of therapists as clients. A qualitative study using a questionnaire survey. *Counselling and Psychotherapy Research, 18*(2), 166–177.

U.S. Census Bureau. (2019). *Race.* Retrieved from https://www.census.gov/topics/population/race/about.html.

Verkuyten, M. (2018). *The social psychology of ethnic identity.* London: Routledge.

Zagefka, H. (2009). The concept of ethnicity in social psychological research: Definitional issues. *International Journal of Intercultural Relations, 33*(3), 228–241.

CHAPTER 5

Cultural Self 2:
Gender and Sex, Disability, and Age

In this chapter, the discussion continues from Chapter 4 on social location concerning major contributors to sense of self and relations with others. It begins with the topics of gender and sex, focusing on the contributions within each area of study and significant findings of research for self-reflection. The chapter concludes with a discussion of the topics of ability and age.

GENDER AND SEX

When you think of gender, what comes to mind? How is gender different from sex? What are the specific aspects of gender and sex that you consider?

Do you see gender and sexual identities as social issues? Political issues? Family issues? Personal issues? How?

Which gender and sexual identities are most and least often represented by therapists in your own experience, as well as by those you have known and worked with? What are the gender and sex compositions of their client bases?

How much do gender and sex matter as a therapist? How is therapist similarity or difference from a client an asset or hindrance?

© The Author(s) 2019   69
J. D. Brown, *Reflective Practice of Counseling and Psychotherapy
in a Diverse Society*, https://doi.org/10.1007/978-3-030-24505-4_5

Definitions of Gender and Sex

Sex is first assigned at the time of birth based on medical considerations such as genitalia, hormones, and chromosomes. (Planned Parenthood, 2019)

Gender refers to the attitudes, feelings, and behaviors that a given culture associates with a person's biological sex. Behavior that is compatible with cultural expectations is gender-normative. (American Psychological Association, 2012)

Sexual orientation is a component of identity that includes a person's sexual and emotional attraction to another person and the behavior or social affiliation that may result from this attraction. A person may be attracted to men, women, both, neither, or to people who are genderqueer, androgynous, or have other gender identities. (American Psychological Association, 2015)

Expressions of Gender and Sex

The gender binary refers to a traditional differentiation of gender into two mutually exclusive categories. Male refers to traditionally masculine traits and female refers to traditionally feminine traits (Hyde, Bigler, Joel, Tate, & van Anders, 2019). Sandra Bem, a pioneer in the concept of gender roles, developed a well-known and still utilized instrument to measure feminine and masculine qualities. Feminine qualities as measured by the short form of Bem instrument (Carver, Vafaei, Guerra, Freire, & Phillips, 2013) include: warm, gentle, affectionate, sympathetic, and sensitive to other's needs. Masculine qualities include leadership abilities, strong personality, dominance, defends own beliefs, and makes decisions quickly. Gender roles include high feminine and high masculine; low masculine high feminine (androgynous), and high masculine and low feminine (undifferentiated). Empirical support of these qualities is associated less with male or female and more to other outcomes. For example, masculine qualities associate with higher rates of illness; the rates of illness occur among males and females with equal frequency but based on the strength of masculine qualities (Carver et al., 2013).

Also, the concept of gender, according to binary models such as the one represented in the Bem Sex Role Inventory, has been found to vary across location and time (Carver et al., 2013). Qualities in this measure speak more to sociocultural context and the timing of the measure. Recent data finds little correspondence between biological sex and gender as measured by the scale. That is, men are no more likely to be masculine than women.

Moreover, fewer and fewer males and females are falling into the traditional categories of masculinity and femininity. Far more common are the categories of androgynous and undifferentiated (Carver et al., 2013). Women, generally, are moving away from feminine qualities and into qualities that reference increased agency and lower communalism to a greater extent than men, and the pattern emerging among postsecondary student populations is less differentiated according to qualities associated with gender (Donnelly & Twenge, 2017).

What do you think about the gender binary? Are masculine and feminine outdated terms? What other terminology is more representative of diversity?

In Canada, updates to one's passport can be voluntary and occur without documentation to indicate female, male, or another gender (Government of Canada, 2019). In the United States, only male and female categories exist, and any change to the gender on one's passport requires medical certification (National Center for Transgender Equality, 2019). What do you see as the benefits and drawbacks of each practice?

Self-Location in Relation to Gender and Sex

Gender includes roles (the norms applied to individuals of a particular sex), identity (how one sees self in relation to masculinity and femininity), relationships (how others treat one based on identity), and how it is institutionalized (distribution of power and authority based on identity) (Smith & Koehoorn, 2016). Gender identity is the sense of self associated with a genderedness within a social and political context where embedded expectations about gender exist (de Graaf, Manjra, Hames, & Zitz, 2018). Gender identity is not necessarily external, so it may not be visible. It is an inherent sense of self. Gender expression is how an individual expresses self in terms of gender (American Psychological

Association, 2012). Gender flexibility affects identity and expression, which can shift (Wood & Eagly, 2015). Gender identities may be affirmed, such as after coming out or having begun a transition process. Identity might be a combination of both genders (bigender, pangender, androgyne), neither gender (genderless, gender-neutral, neutrois, agender), between genders (genderfluid) or another gender entirely (American Psychological Association, 2015).

> How do you identify in relation to gender? What would you indicate as your gender identity? What is central to your sense of self as a gendered person?

Traditionally, assignment at birth has been expected to match the internal sense of self that emerges. Intersex describes a combination of male and female sex characteristics. Variations are multiple and can include ambiguous genitals or internal sex organs, chromosomal issues other than XY (male) and XX (female), male or female genitalia that does not match internal organ or hormonal development during puberty. Historically, medical decisions have been made to surgically alter an intersex child with instructions to caregivers to raise the child according to one or the other. This advice is very problematic as the sexual identity that emerges may be inconsistent with the characteristics retained or stimulated hormonally (MacLaughlin & Donahoe, 2004).

Transgender, Trans or Trans* refers to identity/expression are not the same as assigned sex at birth. Cisgender refers to identity/expression that is the same as assigned sex at birth (American Psychological Association, 2015). There is a very dark history of the treatment of transgender individuals by mental health professionals and the professions of psychiatry and psychology (Dickinson, Cook, Playle, & Hallett, 2012). The mismatch between assigned sex and gender identity was for some time, referred to as gender identity disorder and characterized as a mental illness. Interventions placed individuals into conflict with their gender identity to increase connection with the assigned sex. The harms of this approach were apparent, and it has become recognized that the more proper understanding is gender dysphoria referring to emotional challenges associated with the distress of the mismatch. This understanding is apparent in the American Psychiatric Association's DSM-5 (Beek, Cohen-Kettenis, & Kreukels, 2016). There are many ways that the difference between identity and assigned sex may occur through gender expression, hormonal treatment, and surgical intervention. Passing is presenting as the gender one wants to be seen. There are advantages of safety and affirmation. One potential drawback is being seen as cisgender instead of celebrating transgender.

The American Psychological Association (2019) made a statement about conversion therapy in 2009, and again in 2015 that "Interventions aimed at a fixed outcome, such as gender conformity or heterosexual orientation, including those aimed at changing gender identity, gender expression or sexual orientation, should not be part of behavioral health treatments." What laws exist in your province or state about the practice of conversion therapy? At the time of writing the practice is legal in Canada and the United States, with some exceptions.

Sexual orientation is about with whom one wants to be. Sexuality could be about age, a number of partners, type of activities, sexual consent, intensity, and solitary expressions, but sexual orientation is the most widely known term to describe sexual interest and behavior (Katz-Wise & Hyde, 2015; Rosario & Schrimshaw, 2014; Van Anders, 2015). Sexual orientations are also many and varied. There are several identities associated with sexual orientation (see University of Southern California, 2019). Heterosexual or straight refers to different-gender attraction. Gay typically refers to male to male attraction. Lesbian refers to female to female attraction. Bisexual refers to physical, romantic attraction to more than one gender. Queer refers to not exclusively heterosexual. In LGBTQ, the Q might be queer or questioning. Asexual refers to no physical or romantic attraction. Aromantic refers to no romantic attraction. Androsexual refers to an attraction to masculinity. Bicurious refers to a process of self-understanding and attraction to people of the same or another gender. Demiromantic refers to romantic attraction only after strong physical attraction. Demisexual refers to asexual individuals who have some sexual attraction only after strong emotional attraction. Gynesexual refers to an attraction to femininity. Polyamorous refers to consensual relationships with multiple partners. Skoliosexual refers to attraction to people who are nonbinary, trans, or queer.

Attitudinal and Social Barriers

Consider your own beliefs about gender and sex roles. How will your beliefs as a therapist be evident to a client who identifies differently than you regarding gender identity and sexual orientation.

An illustration of gender roles and behaviors is apparent in the Canadian Labour Force Survey. Existing variables in a database were organized conceptually to create a measure of gender. Sex differences in each of these areas produce a combined score used to define feminine and masculine gender roles (Smith & Koehoorn, 2016).

Do you consider these to be behaviors engaged in by some genders more than others? (1) responsibility for childcare, (2) participation in underrepresented occupations, (3) relative hours of work to partner or spouse, (4) education level relative to partner/spouse, (5) time away from work for family responsibilities. How has participation in these activities changed over time? How do you feel personally about participating in these?

In terms of biological sex, the choices each person has in life depend to a large extent on their chromosomes at birth (Wintemute, 2017). In their review, ways that chromosomes classify or otherwise constrain choices include: (1) work outside of the home and what kind of work, (2) sex characteristics that may be a reason selected for harassment by another, (3) pregnancy and childbirth with associated employment limitations for women, (4) whether one can enter a single-sex location such as institution, bathroom, change room, and (5) in the United Kingdom it determines one's legal sex (Wintemute, 2017). The authors continue to identify the types of discrimination that can occur based on these limitations, including discrimination in childcare allocation, sexual harassment, pregnancy, discrimination against transsexual individuals, gay, lesbian, bisexual, and same-sex couples, as well as discrimination against individuals who appear to violate sex-differentiated dress codes, segregation, and legal classification.

Despite advances in expectations of gendered behaviors, stereotypes based on the gender binary remain prominent (Haines, Deaux, & Lofaro, 2016). Women's roles have remained stereotyped despite changing attitudes about behaviors (Haines et al., 2016). Notwithstanding increasing openness to the participation of women and men in nontraditional areas (e.g. child-rearing, employment), attitudes about what is traditional remain (Haines et al., 2016).

> What stereotypes about men and women have you been exposed to? Which do you resist? Are there any you embrace? Do you believe that the stereotypes you hold as a therapist influence your attitudes, behaviors, judgments, and expectations?

Research concerning the origins of sexual orientation has found repeatedly far more support for the nature side of the nature-nurture issue (de Graaf et al., 2018). Fear and moral judgment are more common among individuals who perceive the nurture of sexual orientation as the stronger contributor (Bailey et al., 2016).

> Is the nature-nurture issue even relevant to the topic of sexual orientation? Why or why not? What are the benefits and drawbacks of viewing sexual orientation as a matter of nature and nurture?

Frequency data on mental health among individuals who identify as lesbian, gay, or bisexual demonstrate differences relative to individuals who identify as heterosexual (Hatzenbuehler, McLaughlin, & Slopen, 2013). Prejudice against individuals who are not cisgender is also very pronounced (Richards & Barker, 2015) and associated with elevated rates of anxiety and depression (de Graaf et al., 2018).

> What can you do as in your practice to take action against fear and prejudice? What could you do to counter negative judgments if prejudicial messages are internalized by a client?

DISABILITY

> When you think of an ability and a disability, what comes to mind? What are the specific aspects of disability that you consider?
>
> Do you see disability as a social issue? Political issue? Family issue? Personal problem? How?
>
> Which disabilities are most and least often represented by therapists in your own experience, as well as by those you have known and worked with? What are the compositions of these client bases?
>
> How much does disability matter as a therapist? How is therapist similarity to the client an asset or hindrance? How could differences between clients and therapists be bridged?

Definitions of Disability

Disability is an evolving concept and that disability results from the interaction between persons with impairments and attitudinal and environmental barriers that hinder their full and active participation in society on an equal basis with others. (United Nations, 2019)

Another definition of disability is *a physical or mental impairment that substantially limits one or more major life activities, a record of such an impairment, or being regarded as having such an impairment* (Americans with Disabilities Act, 1990). Specific examples include *Cancer, Diabetes, HIV, Deafness, Blindness, Limb Damage, Epilepsy* as well as the mental health-related disabilities of *Intellectual Disability, Autism, Major Depressive Disorder and Schizophrenia* (Equal Employment Opportunity Commission, 2011).

Expressions of Disabilities

There are two main perspectives on disability. These include individual and social views (Degener, 2016). Individual views place responsibility for the creation, maintenance, and mitigation of disability on the individual. Problems are caused by factors not associated with the social context. In contrast, societal views place responsibility on the context for the creation, maintenance, and mitigation of disability on the person. From this view, problems that those with disabilities experience are a result of the deficiencies of the societies within which they live (Rothman, 2018).

Western concepts of disability are traceable through modern history. During the Industrial Revolution, discoveries in the sciences contributed to an optimistic view of the potential for human change in response to functional deficits or limited abilities (Albrecht, 1992, pp. 42–46). *The Origin of the Species* reinforced the survival of the fittest and, those best able to adapt would, in their development, produce offspring who are similarly equipped. In this view, adaptation develops through scientific discovery and curative treatment. Species adaptation could also occur by preventing reproduction. Proponents of Eugenics in the nineteenth and twentieth centuries supported reproduction by only the strongest in the interest of human development and social improvement. Those with disabilities were institutionalized, segregated, and sterilized (Rothman, 2018).

Are disabilities an individual experience or contextual construction, or both? Reread the definitions at the start of this section. Does the United Nations definition feel different than the Americans With Disabilities definition? Which resonates more with you? Why? Should any qualities of human variation qualify as a disability? Which ones? In what ways? To what extent?

The conceptual framework for federal census data in Canada defines a disability as a condition lasting six months or more and in one or more of the categories of Seeing, Hearing, Mobility, Flexibility, Dexterity, Pain, Learning, Developmental, Mental, and Memory. The condition needs to cause significant difficulty as well as place activity limitations on that person. Severity scores for adults indicate that 31% have a mild, 19%, a moderate, 23%, a severe, and 27%, a very severe disability (Statistics Canada, 2019).

Do the categories of disability used in the Census have a different tone than diagnoses? Which is more useful in your view? For example, can you have depression but be in remission and have no activity limitations? Does your view change if the "disability" is cancer in remission?

Self-Location in Relation to Disabilities

Persons with disabilities were rejected entirely by some cultures, in others they were outcasts, while in some they were treated as financial liabilities and grudgingly kept alive by their families. In other settings, persons with disabilities were tolerated and treated in incidental ways, while in other cultures they were given respected status and allowed to participate to the fullest extent of their capability. (Munyi, 2012)

In your experience, how are people with physical, intellectual, and emotional disabilities perceived? Are people rejected, outcast, seen as a burden, tolerated, assisted, respected, or revered? Do you have a colleague, friend, or family member with a disability? Do you have a disability? What qualities are central to your sense of self as a person with a disability or as someone without limitations that someone with a disability may have?

Disability as a diagnosable medical condition is deeply engrained in psychology. For example, the outlines obtained from undergraduate psychology courses in the United States focused heavily on cognitive and psychiatric disabilities (Rosa, Bogart, Bonnett, Estill, & Colton, 2016). These disabilities, according to diagnostic criteria, are defined by the absence of something valuable or presence of something undesirable (Brault, 2012). It also assumes that the disability should be treated if possible (Rothman, 2018).

In contrast to the deficit model, the social model of disability places the problems that individuals face on society itself. The fact that individuals with disabilities are disadvantaged provides ample evidence of social injustice and inequity. In this view, impairment can be used to distinguish the condition itself, while disability is the societal response (Degener, 2016). The societal response is evident in the physical environment as well as social values, institutions, and images that are prominent in the culture (Rothman, 2018).

What are or could be the benefits and drawbacks of identifying yourself as a person with a disability? Are there contexts in which it is advantageous to do so? Are there contexts in which it is to your detriment to do so? How would you respond to your therapist who used outdated and diagnostic language to refer to disabilities? How would you respond to a client who told you that your terminology is dated?

Attitudinal and Social Barriers

Research on social aspects of disabilities indicates that discrimination and exclusion are experiences by some individuals who identify as having a disability (e.g. Pownall, Wilson, & Jahoda, 2017). Evidence exists concerning the emotional effects of discrimination, stereotyping, invisibility, and isolation (Rothman, 2018). Lack of personal experience with disability is a significant risk factor for interpersonal comfort, distorted or stereotypical views as well as improper or unfair treatment (Willems, Embregts, Hendriks, & Bosman, 2016).

Consider your own experience with disabilities. How does your own experience influence your comfort in discussing disabilities and impairments, accommodations and advocacy?

Among adults, physical, and sensory disabilities are less stigmatized than intellectual or mental health disabilities (Werner & Araten-Bergman, 2017). Language and social skills differences are also among the more uncomfortable encounters for those with limited personal experience (Lindsay & Cancelliere, 2018). Attitude change is possible, and contact is one means by which this may be promoted (Barr & Bracchitta, 2015).

Medical labels describe conditions as deficits and may have a negative effect through internalized judgments of self and others' reactions (Rothman, 2018). Dependence on healthcare individuals and medical institutions can also reinforce their importance and the language used to characterize the condition and also the individual with the condition. The language is used by the media, as well as in research, professional, and clinical settings. It also has legal significance weighing into its accuracy, meaning, and implications.

As a therapist, how can you address disability from a strength-based perspective? How do you remain cognizant of your attitudes and assumptions about disabilities?

AGE

When you think of age, what comes to mind? What are the specific aspects of age that you consider?

Do you see age as a social issue? Political issue? Family issue? Personal problem? How?

Which ages are most and least often represented by therapists in your own experience, as well as by those you have known and worked with? What are the age compositions of their client bases?

How much does age matter as a therapist? How is therapist similarity to the client an asset? A hindrance?

How is therapist similarity or difference to the client an asset or hindrance? How could differences between clients and therapists be bridged?

Definitions of Age

Age is *the process of developing and maintaining the functional ability that enables wellbeing in older age* (World Health Organization, 2015). Functional ability is *the combination of the intrinsic capacity of the individual, relevant environmental characteristics, and the interactions between the individual and these characteristics* (Beard et al., 2016).

Expressions of Age

A range of views about aging exist. From an evolutionary biology standpoint, aging is a reduction in adaptation over time. It is an age-specific decline in physiological function, reproduction rate, and mortality

(Flatt, 2012). From a social constructivist view, "there are a variety of ways of being old" and little by way of objective indicators (Vincent, 1995). From a cultural perspective, aging is about others' perceptions of what aging is and means.

Successful aging occurs in one of four ways. These include the *amount of activity in which the individual engages, ability to disengage, satisfaction with life, and maturity or integration of personality. The concept of the social system of the individual actor can be used to derive two additional views of successful aging. The first view is the exchange of energy between the individual and the rest of the social system. The second view relates to a judgment concerning the stability of the system, including, especially, the stability of its position concerning autonomy-dependency* (Wirths & Williams, 2017, p. 10).

Do you see aging as having a high or low social value in your family and community? How is aging viewed in the larger society? What assumptions and judgments do you make about those who are older and younger than you?

Self-Location in Relation to Age

How do you identify in terms of your age? Young? Early adulthood? Adulthood? Some other term? What does it mean to you to identify yourself that way? How do you view yourself in comparison to others of different ages or generations? How do you think they view you and others of your age?

Whitbourne and Whitbourne (2010) distinguishes between biological, psychological, and social age. Biology refers to heart, respiration, and endocrine system health. Psychology refers to cognitive and emotional changes. Cognitive changes include memory and learning. Emotional changes refer to emotional awareness and regulation of expression. While there is evidence of cognitive decline, the evidence concerning emotional regulation shows an increase.

Social age refers to milestones in life and to what extent they are met or unmet on time. More specifically, children typically are brought into the family between the ages of 20–40, a first serious relationship is expected to occur during teenage years and young adulthood, entry into the world of work starts during one's 20s and can change with the expectation that there is an advancement of status in each new position. By the mid-late 60s retirement is expected (Whitbourne & Whitbourne, 2010).

Do you agree with the social age expectations listed here? In what ways do your expectations differ? Do you view yourself or others as early, late or on time relative to these milestones? Is it positive or negative or neither to be early or late relative to milestones?

Subjective age is a reflection of how old we feel, appear to others, or want to be. Satisfaction refers to how we feel about our process of aging. In general, aging is experienced positively by those who do not identify as old (Westerhof & Tulle, 2007). These same individuals are also more likely to rate their health as good.

Has anyone ever guessed your age correctly or incorrectly? What age would you like to be seen as? What age would you like to feel like? In what ways do you put effort into being or feeling that age?

Attitudinal and Social Barriers

Consider your own beliefs about these topics and their relevance to your sense of self. Also, how could it be apparent to a client who is the same or different from your age?

> What beliefs do you hold about children, youth, adults, middle-age, older adults? What do you view as typical? What stereotypes do you have about older people? What stereotypes do you expect older adults might hold about someone your age? How can inaccurate attitudes be recognized and addressed in counseling and psychotherapy?

Age-related stereotypes about family (e.g. starting out as a parent in the 20s), leisure (e.g. men going through a mid-life crisis in their 40s), and work (e.g. being career-driven during your 30s) are often internalized by young adults and middle-aged individuals (Kornadt, Voss, & Rothermund, 2015). Older adults face increasingly negative stereotypes about aging (Finkelstein, King, & Voyles, 2015). For example, in a comparison of language used to refer to older individuals in printed sources spanning 200 years, the most prominent stereotypes to emerge concerned medical need, as well as physical and cognitive decline in old age (Ng, Allore, Trentalange, Monin, & Levy, 2015).

> What might you look for as a therapist in a client to indicate a subjective age? What might you look for as a client to indicate the physical, social, and emotional age of your therapist? How much would these ages factor into your judgment of the therapist's ability to help you? Why or why not?

Summary

- Gender identity is the sense of self associated with a genderedness within a particular context containing norms for that gender. Gender identity is who we are, and sexual orientation refers to whom we want to be with.
- There are two major interpretations of disability. Individual models place responsibility for the creation, maintenance, and treatment on the person, while societal models place responsibility on the context.
- Aging may be indicated by physical, intellectual, or emotional changes. Subjective age is how old one feels.

DISCUSSION QUESTIONS

1. Knowing your social locations in relation to gender identity, sexual orientation, disability and age, how far does your comfort level extend? How could you increase your knowledge and experience?
2. What would you expect for the physical structure and contents of your office so that all would feel welcome?
3. How would you respond to a client who is angered because the automatic door is broken, the washrooms are only male or female, a changing table is only in the female washroom, or the signage is in a print that is very small and placed high on the walls?

REFERENCES

Albrecht, G. L. (1992). *The disability business* (Vol. 190). New Delhi: Sage.

American Psychological Association. (2012). Guidelines for psychological practice with lesbian, gay, and bisexual clients. *The American Psychologist, 67*(1), 10.

American Psychological Association. (2015). *Definitions related to sexual orientation and gender diversity in APA documents*. Retrieved from https://www.apa.org/pi/lgbt/resources/sexuality-definitions.pdf.

American Psychological Association. (2019). *APA applauds SAMHSA report calling for end to 'conversion therapy' for youth*. Retrieved from https://www.apa.org/news/press/releases/2015/10/conversion-therapy.

Bailey, J. M., Vasey, P. L., Diamond, L. M., Breedlove, S. M., Vilain, E., & Epprecht, M. (2016). Sexual orientation, controversy, and science. *Psychological Science in the Public Interest, 17*(2), 45–101.

Barr, J. J., & Bracchitta, K. (2015). Attitudes toward individuals with disabilities: The effects of contact with different disability types. *Current Psychology, 34*(2), 223–238.

Beard, J. R., Officer, A., De Carvalho, I. A., Sadana, R., Pot, A. M., Michel, J. P., & Thiyagarajan, J. A. (2016). The World report on ageing and health: A policy framework for healthy ageing. *The Lancet, 387*(10033), 2145–2154.

Beek, T., Cohen-Kettenis, P. T., & Kreukels, B. P. (2016). Gender incongruence/gender dysphoria and its classification history. *International Review of Psychiatry, 28*(1), 5–12.

Brault, M. W. (2012). *Americans with disabilities: 2010* (pp. 1–23). Washington, DC: US Department of Commerce, Economics and Statistics Administration, US Census Bureau.

Carver, L. F., Vafaei, A., Guerra, R., Freire, A., & Phillips, S. P. (2013). Gender differences: Examination of the 12-item Bem Sex Role Inventory (BSRI-12) in an older Brazilian population. *PLoS One, 8*(10), e76356.

Degener, T. (2016). Disability in a human rights context. *Laws, 5*(3), 35.

de Graaf, N. M., Manjra, I. I., Hames, A., & Zitz, C. (2018). Thinking about ethnicity and gender diversity in children and young people. *Clinical Child Psychology and Psychiatry, 24*(2), 291–303. https://doi.org/10.1177/13591 04518805801.

Dickinson, T., Cook, M., Playle, J., & Hallett, C. (2012). Queer' treatments: Giving a voice to former patients who received treatments for their 'sexual deviations. *Journal of Clinical Nursing, 21*(9–10), 1345–1354.

Donnelly, K., & Twenge, J. M. (2017). Masculine and feminine traits on the Bem Sex-Role Inventory, 1993–2012: A cross-temporal meta-analysis. *Sex Roles, 76*(9–10), 556–565.

Equal Employment Opportunity Commission. (2011, March 25, Friday). Rules and regulations. *Federal Register, 76*(58), 16978.

Finkelstein, L. M., King, E. B., & Voyles, E. C. (2015). Age metastereotyping and cross-age workplace interactions: A meta view of age stereotypes at work. *Work, Aging and Retirement, 1*(1), 26–40.

Flatt, T. (2012). A new definition of aging? *Frontiers in Genetics, 3*, 148.

Government of Canada. (2019). *Choose or update the gender identifier on your passport or travel document.* Retrieved from https://www.canada.ca/en/immigration-refugees-citizenship/services/canadian-passports/change-sex.html#document-dont-show-gender.

Haines, E. L., Deaux, K., & Lofaro, N. (2016). The times they are a-changing … or are they not? A comparison of gender stereotypes, 1983–2014. *Psychology of Women Quarterly, 40*(3), 353–363.

Hatzenbuehler, M. L., McLaughlin, K. A., & Slopen, N. (2013). Sexual orientation disparities in cardiovascular biomarkers among young adults. *American Journal of Preventive Medicine, 44*(6), 612–621.

Hyde, J. S., Bigler, R. S., Joel, D., Tate, C. C., & van Anders, S. M. (2019). The future of sex and gender in psychology: Five challenges to the gender binary. *American Psychologist, 74*(2), 171.

Katz-Wise, S. L., & Hyde, J. S. (2015). Sexual fluidity and related attitudes and beliefs among young adults with a same-gender orientation. *Archives of Sexual Behavior, 44*(5), 1459–1470.

Kornadt, A. E., Voss, P., & Rothermund, K. (2015). Hope for the best, prepare for the worst? Future self- views and preparation for age-related changes. *Psychology and Aging, 30*(4), 967.

Lindsay, S., & Cancelliere, S. (2018). A model for developing disability confidence. *Disability and Rehabilitation, 40*(18), 2122–2130.

MacLaughlin, D. T., & Donahoe, P. K. (2004). Sex determination and differentiation. *New England Journal of Medicine, 350*(4), 367–378.

Munyi, C. W. (2012). Past and present perceptions towards disability: A historical perspective. *Disability Studies Quarterly, 32*(2), 1–11.

National Center for Transgender Equality. (2019). *Can I get a passport with my current gender?* Retrieved from https://transequality.org/know-your-rights/passports.

Ng, R., Allore, H. G., Trentalange, M., Monin, J. K., & Levy, B. R. (2015). Increasing negativity of age stereotypes across 200 years: Evidence from a database of 400 million words. *PLoS One, 10*(2), e0117086.

Planned Parenthood. (2019). *Gender and gender identity.* Retrieved from https://www.plannedparenthood.org/learn/sexual-orientation-gender/gender-gender-identity.

Pownall, J., Wilson, S., & Jahoda, A. (2017). Health knowledge and the impact of social exclusion on young people with intellectual disabilities. *Journal of Applied Research in Intellectual Disabilities,* 1–10.

Richards, C., & Barker, M. J. (Eds.). (2015). *The Palgrave handbook of the psychology of sexuality and gender.* Berlin: Springer.

Rosa, N. M., Bogart, K. R., Bonnett, A. K., Estill, M. C., & Colton, C. E. (2016). Teaching about disability in psychology: An analysis of disability curricula in US undergraduate psychology programs. *Teaching of Psychology, 43*(1), 59–62.

Rosario, M., & Schrimshaw, E. W. (2014). Theories and etiologies of sexual orientation. In D. L. Tolman & L. M. Diamond (Eds.), *APA handbook of sexuality and psychology. Volume 1: Person-based approaches.* Washington, DC: American Psychological Association.

Rothman, J. (2018). *Social work practice across disability.* New York: Routledge.

Smith, P. M., & Koehoorn, M. (2016). Measuring gender when you don't have a gender measure: Constructing a gender index using survey data. *International Journal for Equity in Health, 15*(1), 82.

Statistics Canada. (2019). *Disabilities in Canada.* https://www150.statcan.gc.ca/n1/pub/75-006-x/2014001/article/14115-eng.htm.

The Americans with Disabilities Act. (1990). *ADA acronyms & abbreviations.* https://adata.org/acronyms-abbreviations.

United Nations. (2019). *Department of economic and social affairs: Disability.* Retrieved September 13 from: https://www.un.org/development/desa/disabilities/convention-on-the-rights-of-persons-with-disabilities/preamble.html.

University of Southern California. (2019). *LGBT resource centre.* Retrieved from https://lgbtrc.usc.edu/education/terminology/.

Van Anders, S. M. (2015). Beyond sexual orientation: Integrating gender/sex and diverse sexualities via sexual configurations theory. *Archives of Sexual Behavior, 44*(5), 1177–1213.

Vincent, J. (1995). *Inequality and old age.* London: UCL Press.

Werner, S., & Araten-Bergman, T. (2017). Social workers' stigmatic perceptions of individuals with disabilities: A focus on three disabilities. *Journal of Mental Health Research in Intellectual Disabilities, 10*(2), 93–107.

Westerhof, G. J., & Tulle, E. (2007). Meanings of ageing and old age: Discursive contexts, social attitudes and personal identities. In J. Bond, S. Peace, F. Dittmann-Kohli, & G. J. Westerhof (Eds.), *Ageing in society* (pp. 235–254). London: Sage.

Whitbourne, S. K., & Whitbourne, S. B. (2010). *Adult development and aging: Biopsychosocial perspectives*. Hoboken, NJ: Wiley.

Willems, A. P. A. M., Embregts, P. J. C. M., Hendriks, L., & Bosman, A. (2016). Towards a framework in interaction training for staff working with clients with intellectual disabilities and challenging behaviour. *Journal of Intellectual Disability Research, 60*(2), 134–148.

Wintemute, R. (2017). Recognising new kinds of direct sex discrimination: Transsexualism, sexual orientation and dress codes. In N. Bamforth (Ed.), *Sexual orientation and rights* (pp. 265–290). London: Routledge.

Wirths, C. G., & Williams, R. A. (2017). *Lives through the years: Styles of life and successful aging*. New York: Routledge.

Wood, W., & Eagly, A. H. (2015). Two traditions of research on gender identity. *Sex Roles, 73*(11–12), 461–473.

World Health Organization. (2015). *World report on ageing and health*. Retrieved from http://www.who.int/ageing/events/world-report-2015-launch/en/.

CHAPTER 6

Intersections and Power

SOCIAL LOCATION

Social location refers to "the groups people belong to because of their place or position in history and society. All people have a social location that is defined by their gender, race, social class, age, ability, religion, sexual orientation, and geographic location. Each group membership confers a certain set of social roles and rules, power, and privilege (or lack of), which heavily influence our identity" (University of Victoria, 2019). Social location is about group membership, and identity is a subjective sense of self. Review Fig. 6.1 and edit the descriptors that contribute to your sense of identity.

Take a moment to insert specific qualities in Fig. 6.2 using the descriptors in Fig. 6.1 as a guide. Once you have listed the qualities in Fig. 6.2, circle those that are the most important to your sense of self. Draw a line through those that are the least important to your sense of self. What does this activity say about you? How do you describe yourself to others? How do others perceive you?

© The Author(s) 2019
J. D. Brown, *Reflective Practice of Counseling and Psychotherapy in a Diverse Society*, https://doi.org/10.1007/978-3-030-24505-4_6

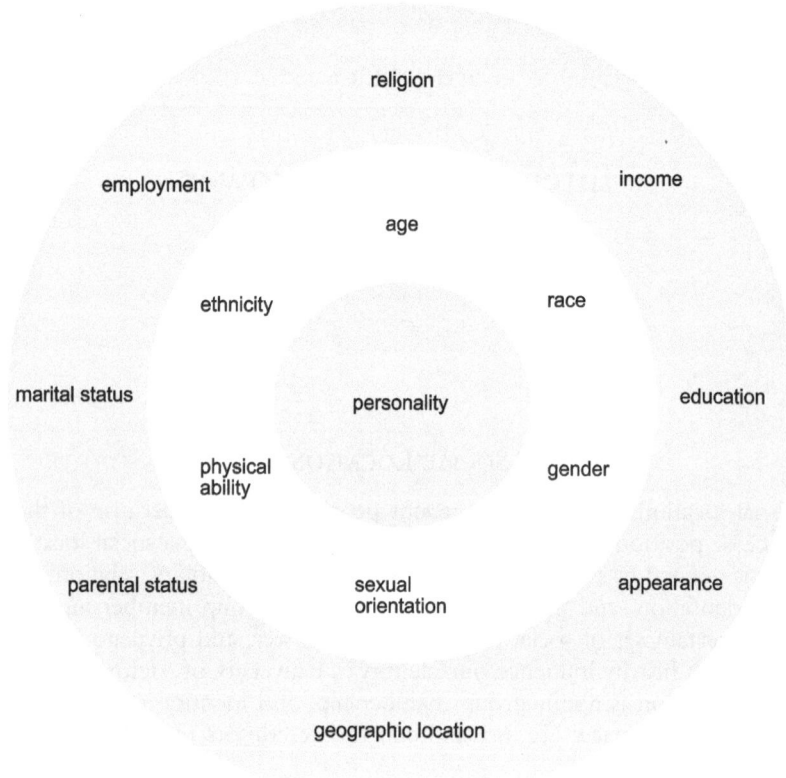

Fig. 6.1 Social locations

IDENTITY

Identity is the internal sense and identification of oneself (Leary & Tangney, 2011). Identity is apparent in beliefs and values, thoughts, and behavior, as well as meaning and purpose (Leary & Tangney, 2011). While we generally approach situations in an identity-consistent manner (e.g. what we notice, experience, and respond to, as well as how we act and think), we are also capable of functioning in identity-inconsistent ways (Leary & Tangney, 2011).

Fig. 6.2 Identity

Three main types of identity include personal, social, and role. Personal identity refers to the self in development (Stryker & Burke, 2000). It includes descriptive qualities of the individual as well as one's feelings about them. Social identity is the sense of self-in-relation that connects with group membership (Tajfel, 1981). It may vary across contexts and situations. Finally, role identity is associated with a particular function. Roles are forms of social identity insofar as they require another person or persons in order to function in that role (e.g. the role of a parent requires a child) (Leary & Tangney, 2011).

Stability of identity across time and contexts is necessary to maintain an accurate and meaningful sense of self (Stryker & Burke, 2000). However, it has been argued that it is the adaptability to change that matters (Leary & Tangney, 2011).

How have the qualities in Fig. 6.2 changed or remained constant? Has their importance changed? What do you attribute the change or consistency to?

Identity Development

Identity progresses from lower to more advanced levels of development. Erik Eriksen's theory remains influential (Hoover, 2004). Although identity is said to develop only during adolescence, the development that occurs before and after reflects both building blocks and potential outcomes of identity formation.

In Trust vs. Mistrust, the unpredictability of experience filters through a consistent caregiver that, when successful, leads to a sense of hope. If unsuccessful, the outcome is fear. In Autonomy vs. Shame, the desire to become more active in exploration is met with increasing independence; the outcome is will. If met with control, inadequacy is the result. If caregivers embolden initiative in the following stage, Initiative vs. Guilt, the result is a sense of purpose. Industry vs. Inferiority requires the exercise of skills learned as well as encouragement and deserved praise, with feelings of competency as the result.

Between the ages of 12 and 18, identity is developed. Identity develops as a result of active exploration and trying on of different identities. The experimentation process is essential, and arrival at a clear sense of self is important to continue healthy development. When this does not happen, the result is confusion and alienation. In Intimacy vs. Isolation, young adults are expected to develop intimate relationships, and if so, love is the resulting virtue. Generativity vs. Stagnation is the next stage that describes the felt need for making a difference in the community through one's actions. Feeling connected to their community, individuals who are successful in this stage develop care. Finally, in Ego Integrity vs. Despair self-acceptance and reflection on a meaningful life lead to the virtue of wisdom (McLeod, 2013).

James Marcia (1993) further developed Eriksen's identity stage into a more detailed model. He added the components of exploration and commitment. In exploration, there is an active search and acting as though one is a particular self. In commitment, there is a sense of clarity and purpose reflected in the decision made. There are four corresponding identity statuses. Achievement is the commitment to identity after a period of exploration. Foreclosure is the commitment to an identity without any exploration. The moratorium is no commitment but active exploration. Finally, diffusion is neither exploration nor commitment (Crocetti & Salmela-Aro, 2018). Subsequent meta-analytic research has found support for the general notion of identity development during adolescence, and identity status tends to occur from diffusion to foreclosure, and moratorium to achievement (Meeus, 2018).

The question of how identity forms is a more recent undertaking. The type and intensity of commitment and exploration are factors (Crocetti & Salmela-Aro, 2018). Commitment separates into commitment making and identification with commitment. Exploration includes past exploration and present exploration. In this model, the process of identity formation occurs before and after adolescence through ongoing consideration of one's commitments and taking on new commitments.

Development of Racial Identity

Racial identity occurs developmentally. The frequently identified models include Cross People of Color Racial Identity Model (Cross, 1985), Poston's Biracial Identity Development (Poston, 1990), and Helms' White Racial Identity Model (Helms, 1990).

In the People of Color Racial Identity Model (Cross, 1985) there are five stages, including pre-encounter, encounter, immersion/emersion, internalization, and internalization/commitment. In pre-encounter distancing from one's race is done in order to associate with those of the majority race. The encounter begins with the realization that one is not a member and cannot be a member of the majority race and that they are affected by racism. Immersion/emersion marks a distancing from members of the majority race and increasing affiliations with one's race through community connections and embracing symbols that exemplify that affiliation.

Internalization is the achievement of a healthy racial identity from which connecting with members of the majority race is possible, and internalization/commitment is understanding of race as differentiating but not the only way.

In Biracial Identity Development (Poston, 1990) there are five stages including personal identity, choice of group characterization, enmeshment/denial, appreciation, and integration. Personal identity is a sense of self created from interacting with family and friends as well as other external influences. The pressure to select an ethnic or racial group over another occurs as a choice of group characterization. Enmeshment/denial refers to a guilt response after leaving one group, feeling subsequent pressure to adopt both, and the rationalization that there are only similarities between them. Appreciation refers to newfound recognition of the group that had a lesser emphasis in earlier development and desire to learn more about it. Finally, in integration, the individual can identify with one race as well as appreciate how they also have another identity.

There are two major stages in the White Racial Identity Model (Helms, 1990), including the Abandonment of Racism and Evolution of a Non-Racist Identity. Abandonment of Racism includes three substages of contact (race is only a physical quality), disintegration (can begin to see racism in self) and reintegration (denial of racism in self and others). In Evolution of a Non-Racist Identity, the substages include pseudo-independence (interested but superficial), immersion/emersion (find a way to understand what it means to be White) and autonomy (accepting one's Whiteness and role in racism).

INTERSECTIONALITY

The concept of intersectionality has its origins in Black feminism. Crenshaw (1988) first wrote about intersectionality to highlight the ways that race, class, and gender interact and affect how women of color experience oppression. For example, at times, a Black woman may have similar experiences to Black men, but other times, as a woman who is also Black and as well as a Black woman. The latter two conditions are double discrimination and double jeopardy, respectively (Cole, 2009). Critical aspects of intersectionality include an explicit recognition of the context, advantage and disadvantage, and co-occurring experiences, as well as the centrality of power in relationships (Carastathis, 2016).

Three types of intersectionality include voice, relational, and anti-categorical (Choo & Ferree, 2010). From an anti-categorical perspective, categories cannot reflect the diversity of experience. Categories are themselves problematic because they oversimplify and essentialize. In the case of racialized gender, the two categories suggest a simplicity that is, in reality, far more detailed and nuanced. The categories do an injustice to those it is intended to describe. From a voice perspective, the representation of a particular group is paramount. The focus is on a single category at a particular point of intersection and in a particular setting. The purpose is to elevate the voice of a particular group (Nash, 2008). From a relational perspective, it is the interaction between statuses represented by groups that are the focus. So, for example, how is gender racialized? Assuming that changes occur over time and context, the analysis is always in motion.

Identities and Intersections

Identity may be described, at least to some extent, by the intersecting locations. While the degree to which these intersections reflect any one person's experience varies considerably, they are a useful starting point for learning about self and comparison to others, as well as power within the therapeutic relationship. Identities are multiple and complex, generally consistent, but to some extent dependent on the context which produces and regulates them (Levine-Rasky, 2011).

Identities and intersections must not represent the person (Carastathis, 2016). It is equally essential to avoid overgeneralizations. For example, (a) all women experience equal oppression, (b) the oppression is present to the same extent and the same way in every context, (c) the experience of womanhood is the same internally and subjectively as it is expressed, and (d) the oppression necessarily causes a lack of fulfillment or well-being (Nash, 2008).

There is always a hierarchy in a relationship. However, it can shift. For example, the same person can feel differently about self throughout a conversation, about the conversation itself relative to other relationships, as well as relationships more generally. Few of us are purely advantaged or disadvantaged (Carastathis, 2016). The context impacts on the relationships within it (Samuels & Ross-Sheriff, 2008).

Consider Table 6.1. In the cells are possible labels for advantaged and disadvantage. For each social location, identify what is typical in (1) society, (2) your community, and (3) your profession? Then identify your social location and whether it reflects privilege or disadvantage.

Table 6.1   Identity matrices

	Class	Race and ethnicity	Gender and sex	Ability	Age
Society					
Privileged					
Disadvantaged					
My location					
Community					
Privileged					
Disadvantaged					
Profession					
Privileged					
Disadvantaged					

> Which intersections are most and least often represented in your own experience as a therapist, as well as those you have known and worked with? What benefits and challenges have you experienced and anticipate concerning differences between yourself and clients? Which will be most and least beneficial and challenging? Why?

POWER

Different bases of power exist (Homan, 2010). Information includes access to relevant data that is public or private, global or local. Money is another source of power, which could include financial institutions as well as businesses that have financial holdings. Laws are legal requirements to conform in specific ways that have legal consequences. Constituencies are groups within a broader community who exercise their influence. Energy and natural resources refer to existing physical characteristics that have economic, cultural, social, or political value. Goods and services refer to sources of power that are harvested, created, or developed that can be bought and sold. Network participation as a source of power includes members of relevant social networks and interconnections between individuals and groups that act cohesively. Families have power through their history of collaborations and achievements. Illegal actions, those that run counter to the laws in place, are also a source of power. Status occupations, including professionals, cultural, or religious leaders, have positions of power.

It has been said that "there is no center without a border, no privilege without oppression" (Levine-Rasky, 2011). Power is expressed in public policies (determining who gets what and when), social hierarchies (determining whom within organizations and communities has more influence), culturally (determining the language and ways that hierarchies are legitimized), and interpersonally (determining how individuals experience their own and other's identities) (Collins, 2019).

> How do you view social, economic, and political power? Positively? Negatively? Both positive and negative? In what ways? Neither positive or negative? Why?

Personal Power

Freud and Adler's theories of development and personality speak to power as dominance, while Maslow and Horney characterize personal power as a positive development and necessary for self-actualization. Cognitive psychology includes many constructs measuring personal power, such as competence and mastery (White, 1959) personal causation (DeCharms, 1972), autonomy (Heider's, 2013), agency (Ryan & Deci, 2000), locus of control (Rotter, 1966), illusions of control (Taylor & Brown, 1988), learned helplessness (Maier & Seligman, 1976), and self-efficacy (Bandura, 1977).

> How do you view personal power? Is it positive? Negative? Both positive and negative? In what ways? Neither positive or negative? Why?

Different models of personal power exist. Steiner's (2017) model includes standing one's ground, knowledge, control, communication, passion, love, and transcendence. Other bases include awareness, values, skills, information, and purpose (Beetham, 2013). Awareness is what one brings of self into the situation. Values refer to principles underlying decisions and actions. Skills are specialized abilities and instruments that develop through training and experience. Information is the knowledge held about the topic at hand.

One who feels powerful can recognize rewards (Galinsky et al., 2013) and is willing to take chances (Keltner, 2003). Personal power allows for the expression of authenticity and dissenting opinions (Keltner et al., 2003). However, it does so out of self-focus, willingness to cut corners to make decisions, as well as potentially reduced recognition of others' opinions, and use of others for personal gain (Galinsky et al., 2008).

Powerlessness is associated with greater awareness of potential threats and lower risk-taking (Keltner, 2003; Keltner et al., 2003). In contrast to feeling powerful, feeling powerless results in inhibition and safe-conduct (Galinsky et al., 2013), leading to an agreement and following norms. There is more of a problem-focus and self-preservation orientation with safety as a primary concern affecting how one thinks acts and feels (Richman & Lattanner, 2014).

Which of these types of personal power are most and least influential? Which are most credible to you? Why? Put yourself in the role of one who reports experiencing several forms of disadvantage and reconsider these types of power. At what point does the helpful use of power become an abuse of power? As a therapist, how would you recognize this? What would you do? As a client, how would you recognize and feel if a therapist was abusing their power? What would you do?

Therapist Power

The power that counselors and psychotherapists have is part of the organizational and professional culture within which they work. This power can exist in different ways, such as reward, coercive, legitimate, referent, expert, and informational (Pierro, Raven, Amato, & Bélanger, 2013). Coercion is the effort to gain compliance through force. Reward power is the ability to provide something tangible or to withdraw it. Legitimate power is a socially sanctioned process. Referent power refers to associations. Expert power rests on knowledge or skills. Informational power is the means to reserve or share information.

Power as counselors and psychotherapists includes the privilege bestowed on one as a professional, within a structure that protects that role, within a society that legitimizes that position with specific expertise, skills, and status (Guilfoyle, 2003).

There are many examples of power in the therapeutic relationship (Hernández & McDowell, 2010). A list of topics representing power in therapy (Zur, 2019) includes: who asks questions, therapist self-disclosure, mystery of what therapy is, specialized knowledge, labeling, having a client one on one, set the parameters, clients need something, and therapists have that something, use of victim language, jargon, and language, as well as taking notes.

Empowerment is the enhancement of personal power. Its history is in liberation psychology (Freire, 1970). It offers a purpose for capitalizing on client strengths. For example, clients can access or already possess resources based on their group memberships. Families, networks, and constituencies can be equally important sources of power. Personal sources of power exist within all of us. Despite initial disadvantages clients face in the therapeutic relationship, each possesses influence with others (Thibaut & Kelley, 1959).

Zur (2019) has offered a list of topics that may represent a shift of power in the therapeutic relationship over time. Some of these include more clarity about the process, informed consent, not talking, doing homework, attending, coming late or leaving early, not paying, taking notes or recording sessions, different seating arrangements, touch or gifts, suicidal gestures or threats, complaints to the regulating body.

Different therapies emphasize different degrees of the power imbalance between therapist and client. Which do you see as your most comfortable starting place in terms of a balance between therapist and client? Therapist > Client, Client > Therapist, Client = Therapist? What are the potential advantages and disadvantages of this? Is a shift necessary at times or should the distribution of power remain consistent with a particular client? Why or why not?

Differential Access

There are several reasons why counseling and psychotherapy services may not be utilized. Issues reported in the literature include stigma, fears about what treatment is, fear of emotion, expected benefits/risks, self-disclosure, norms, and self-esteem (Blake, 2008). Ethnic considerations concern the degree to which therapy and seeing a therapist are inconsistent with culture. For example, concerns may include privacy, someone outside family/church knowing one's personal information, avoidance rather than disclosure is a preferred way to handle problems, the existence of problems is taboo, the value of prayer over treatment, and potential of losing face (Watkins, 2017). The greater the experience of oppression and discrimination, the lower the likelihood of utilizing health and mental health care, including counseling and psychotherapy (Vogel, Wester, & Larson, 2007).

One approach to make counseling and psychotherapy more inclusive is to consider the barriers to service. Barriers include availability, accessibility, acceptability, appropriateness, and adequacy (Gallagher & Truglio-Londrigan, 2004). Availability concerns whether the service is available. Acceptability refers to whether potential clients feel that they can use the services. Affordability includes the actual and perceived costs of accessing the service. Appropriateness is whether the service is the right kind of service. Adequacy is about how comprehensive the service is needed to be and is.

> Consider the settings where you have observed, been employed or practiced as a therapist. Who were the clients? Who were the therapists? Now consider whom you did not see as clients. Who are those individuals? Who was not served by the agency? Why do you think that was the case?

Differential Effectiveness

Common factors indicate which therapist is most appropriate and effective for which client. However, there has been relatively little attention to the circumstances of life outside of therapy and extent to which oppression and discrimination, as well as other social, political, and economic conditions, limit the effectiveness of counseling and psychotherapy

(Messer, 2009). Client factors can be understood to include internal (what is present during the therapy encounter) as well as external (what is present for a client outside of the therapeutic encounter). Social support is one understudied but vital component (Feeney & Collins, 2015).

Whom do you think the types of counseling and psychotherapy you have observed or engaged in are best suited for? What is the cultural makeup of the clients who are most likely to be successful in therapy? What is the cultural makeup of the clients who are least likely to be successful in therapy? Why do you think that is the case? What does it say about the therapy? The therapist? The setting?

Summary

- Identity may be broadly defined as how one recognizes and understands themselves.
- Crenshaw first wrote about intersectionality to highlight the ways that race, class, and gender affect the ways that women of color experience oppression.
- Power is always present in the networking of identities and other identities within a particular place and time.
- Empowerment is rooted in liberation psychology. It offers a purpose for capitalizing on the power that a client possesses to enhance it.

Discussion Questions

1. Errors that therapists may make concerning identity could be oversimplification, overgeneralizing, essentializing, and assimilationism (Shin, 2015). Has this ever happened to you? In what context and ways? How did you respond?
2. In what contexts do you feel the most disadvantaged? School, work, home, community? Where do you feel the most privileged? Why? What will it be like to work with a client who has a sense of superiority to you by virtue of their combination of intersecting identities?
3. Is it possible as a therapist to evenly split power with a client? Is it desirable? Is it ethical?

REFERENCES

Bandura, A. (1977). Self-efficacy: Toward a unifying theory of behavioral change. *Psychological Review, 84*(2), 191–215.

Beetham, D. (2013). *The legitimation of power*. Basingstoke: Macmillan International Higher Education.

Blake, J. P. (2008). *Psychological distress, masculinity ideology, and self-threat: A model of men's attitudes toward help seeking*. New York: Fordham University.

Carastathis, A. (2016). *Intersectionality: Origins, contestations, horizons*. Lincoln, NE: University of Nebraska Press.

Choo, H. Y., & Ferree, M. M. (2010). Practicing intersectionality in sociological research: A critical analysis of inclusions, interactions, and institutions in the study of inequalities. *Sociological Theory, 28*(2), 129–149.

Cole, E. R. (2009). Intersectionality and research in psychology. *American Psychologist, 64*(3), 170.

Collins, P. H. (2019). The difference that power makes: Intersectionality and participatory democracy. In O. Hankivsky & J. S. Jordan-Zachery (Eds.), *The Palgrave handbook of intersectionality in public policy* (pp. 167–192). Cham: Palgrave Macmillan.

Crenshaw, K. W. (1988). Race, reform, and retrenchment: Transformation and legitimation in antidiscrimination law. *Harvard Law Review, 101,* 1331–1387.

Crocetti, E., & Salmela-Aro, K. (2018). The multifaceted nature of identity toward integrative perspectives on processes, pathways, and contexts. *European Psychologist, 23*(4), 273–277.

Cross, W. E. (1985). Black identity: Rediscovering the distinction between personal identity and reference group orientation. In M. B. Spencer, G. K. Brookins, & W. R. Allen (Eds.), *Beginnings: The social and affective development of Black children* (pp. 155–171). Hillsdale, NJ: Lawrence Erlbaum.

Decharms, R. (1972). Personal causation training in the schools. *Journal of Applied Social Psychology, 2*(2), 95–113.

Feeney, B. C., & Collins, N. L. (2015). A new look at social support: A theoretical perspective on thriving through relationships. *Personality and Social Psychology Review, 19*(2), 113–147.

Freire, P. (1970). *Pedagogy of the oppressed* (M. B. Ramos, Trans.). New York: Continuum.

Galinsky, A. D., Magee, J. C., Gruenfeld, D. H., Whitson, J. A., & Liljenquist, K. A. (2008). Power reduces the press of the situation: Implications for creativity, conformity, and dissonance. *Journal of Personality and Social Psychology, 95*(6), 1450.

Galinsky, A. D., Wang, C. S., Whitson, J. A., Anicich, E. M., Hugenberg, K., & Bodenhausen, G. V. (2013). The reappropriation of stigmatizing labels: The reciprocal relationship between power and self-labeling. *Psychological Science, 24*(10), 2020–2029.

Gallagher, L. P., & Truglio-Londrigan, M. (2004). Using the "Seven A's" assessment tool for developing competency in case management. *The Journal of the New York State Nurses' Association, 35*(1), 26–31.

Guilfoyle, M. (2003). Dialogue and power: A critical analysis of power in dialogical therapy. *Family Process, 42*(3), 331–343.

Heider, F. (2013). *The psychology of interpersonal relations*. London: Psychology Press.

Helms, J. E. (1990). *Black and white racial identity: Theory, research, and practice*. New York: Greenwood Press.

Hernández, P., & McDowell, T. (2010). Intersectionality, power, and relational safety in context: Key concepts in clinical supervision. *Training and Education in Professional Psychology, 4*(1), 29.

Homan, M. S. (2010). *Promoting community change: Making it happen in the real world*. Toronto: Nelson Education.

Hoover, K. (Ed.). (2004). *The future of identity: Centennial reflections on the legacy of Erik Erikson*. Lanham: Lexington Books.

Richman, L. S., & Lattanner, M. R. (2014). Self-regulatory processes underlying structural stigma and health. *Social Science and Medicine, 103*, 94–100.

Keltner, D. (2003). Expression and the course of life. *Annals of the New York Academy of Sciences, 1000*(1), 222–243.

Keltner, D., Gruenfeld, D. H., & Anderson, C. (2003). Power, approach, and inhibition. *Psychological Review, 110*(2), 265.

Leary, M. R., & Tangney, J. P. (Eds.). (2011). *Handbook of self and identity*. London: Guilford Press.

Levine-Rasky, C. (2011). Intersectionality theory applied to whiteness and middle-classness. *Social Identities, 17*(2), 239–253.

Maier, S. F., & Seligman, M. E. (1976). Learned helplessness: theory and evidence. *Journal of Experimental Psychology: General, 105*(1), 3.

Marcia, J. E. (1993). The ego identity status approach to ego identity. In J. E. Marcia, A. S. Waterman, D. R. Matteson, S. L. Archer, & J. L. Orlofsky (Eds.), *Ego identity* (pp. 3–21). New York, NY: Springer.

McLeod, S. A. (2013). *Erik Erikson*. Retrieved March 9, 2017.

Meeus, W. (2018). The identity status continuum revisited. *European Psychologist, 23*, 289–299.

Messer, S. B. (2009). Common factors in psychotherapy: Three perspectives. *Applied and Preventive Psychology, 13*(1–4), 22–23.

Nash, J. C. (2008). Re-thinking intersectionality. *Feminist Review, 89*(1), 1–15.

Pierro, A., Raven, B. H., Amato, C., & Bélanger, J. J. (2013). Bases of social power, leadership styles, and organizational commitment. *International Journal of Psychology, 48*(6), 1122–1134.

Poston, W. C. (1990). The biracial identity development model: A needed addition. *Journal of Counseling & Development, 69*(2), 152–155.

White, Robert W. (1959). Motivation reconsidered: The concept of competence. *Psychological Review, 66*(5), 297–333.

Rotter, J. (1966). Generalized expectancies for internal versus external control of reinforcement. *Psychological Monographs: General and Applied, 80*(1), 1–28.

Ryan, R. M., & Deci, E. L. (2000). Self-determination theory and the facilitation of intrinsic motivation, social development, and well-being. *American Psychologist, 55*, 68–78.

Samuels, G. M., & Ross-Sheriff, F. (2008). Identity, oppression, and power: Feminisms and intersectionality theory. *AFFILIA: The Journal of Women and Social Work, 23*, 5–9.

Shin, R. Q. (2015). The application of critical consciousness and intersectionality as tools for decolonizing racial/ethnic identity development models in the fields of counseling and psychology. In R. D. Goodman & P. C. Gorski (Eds.), *Decolonizing "multicultural" counseling through social justice* (pp. 11–22). New York, NY: Springer.

Steiner, C. M. (2017). The seven sources of power: An alternative to authority. *Transactional Analysis Journal, 17*(3), 102–104.

Stryker, S., & Burke, P. J. (2000). The past, present, and future of an identity theory. *Social Psychology Quarterly, 63*, 284–297.

Tajfel, H. (1981). *Human groups and social categories: Studies in social psychology.* Cambridge: CUP Archive.

Taylor, S. E., & Brown, J. D. (1988). Illusion and well-being: A social psychological perspective on mental health. *Psychological Bulletin, 103*(2), 193.

Thibaut, J. W., & Kelley, H. H. (1959). Power and dependence. *The Social Psychology of Groups, 7*, 100–125.

University of Victoria. (2019). *Cultural safety.* Retrieved July 31, from https://web2.uvcs.uvic.ca/courses/csafety/mod2/glossary.htm#Q.

Vogel, D. L., Wester, S. R., & Larson, L. M. (2007). Avoidance of counseling: Psychological factors that inhibit seeking help. *Journal of Counseling & Development, 85*(4), 410–422.

Watkins, T. A. (2017). *"We Don't Talk about That": Mental health promotion by parents in African American communities* (Doctoral diss.).

Zur, O. (2019). *Power in psychotherapy and counseling.* Retrieved from https://www.zurinstitute.com/power-in-therapy/.

Emotions and Countertransference

EMOTIONS

References to emotions are evident within Western and Eastern philosophical and religious traditions. The earliest record is that of Hindu philosophers (Barrett, Lewis, & Haviland-Jones, 2016). Originally written in Sanskrit, these states of mind have been roughly translated into English as rati (passion), hiisa (happy), soka (sadness), krodha (anger), bhaya (fear), utsiiha (determination), jugupsii (disgust), vismaya (excitement), and sama (calm). One well known contemporary Western model of emotion includes ecstasy, admiration, terror, amazement, grief, loathing, rage, and vigilance (Plutchik, 1997). Similarities and differences between these two, include convergence on the emotions of passion and ecstasy, sadness and grief, fear and terror, disgust and loathing, as well as rage and anger. Not only are the types of emotion evidenced in early writings, but their expression as well. The Natya Shastra is a manual of dramatic art written in about 200 BC. It includes a chapter on the causes and consequences of the original emotion states and their representation in theater (Barrett et al., 2016). Readers are advised to consider various forms of expression, including what appears in one's face, voice, action, physiological response, and posture.

More recent analyses of emotional experience and expression across cultures integrate the anthropological and psychological work of Horton (2006 in Shwder, Haidt, Horton, & Joseph, 2008). This analysis

© The Author(s) 2019
J. D. Brown, *Reflective Practice of Counseling and Psychotherapy in a Diverse Society*, https://doi.org/10.1007/978-3-030-24505-4_7

produced common elements of emotion. These include observable phys-ical evidence, affect, conditions that produce the emotion, significance, social judgment, management of emotion, expression to others, and response to others' expressions (Barrett et al., 2016).

Emotions connect with values. That is, some values are emotions, and those emotions have cultural, moral, and religious significance. For example, Al-Ghazali's typology of virtues included wisdom, courage, and temperance (Sherif, 1975). Courage, it was thought, included the emotions of intrepidity, endurance, and amiability. Temperance included modesty, patience, contentment, cheerfulness, tranquility, and righteous indignation. Recent studies of these virtues among a sample of individ-uals identifying themselves as Muslims in the United States (Joseph, 2001) found a great deal of similarity between the virtues listed by Al-Ghazali and those of contemporary significance. The emotions listed as virtues included optimism and patience, self-control and modesty, courage, humility, gentleness, forbearance, and forgiveness. Additional emotions included the love of others, good relations with kin, compas-sion, and gratitude (Barrett et al., 2016).

Categories of Emotions

Emotions are adaptive responses to circumstances that promote sur-vival (Plutchik, 1997). They are evolutionary. Also, there are only a few primary emotions from which other emotions derive (Demoulin et al., 2004; Thoits, 1989). Although the intensity of experience and expres-sion vary, the fundamental structure is believed to be universal (Kohler et al., 2004).

A recent study that used emotional vocabulary from existing liter-ature and represented these using video vignettes found a total of 27 different emotions. The emotion vocabulary used is listed in the follow-ing table and represented in 2000 videos. The resulting emotions can be said to have a great deal of agreement on their presence and distinc-tive nonverbal signals. The emotions include Admiration, Adoration, Aesthetic appreciation, Amusement, Anger, Anxiety, Awe, Awkwardness, Boredom, Calmness, Confusion, Craving, Disgust, Empathic pain, Entrancement, Excitement, Fear, Horror, Interest, Joy, Nostalgia, Relief, Romance, Sadness, Satisfaction, Sexual Desire, and Surprise (Cowen & Keltner, 2017).

From the list in Box 7.1 circle all that you recognize as experiencing yourself during the past week and month. What is most familiar to you? Which on the list are unfamiliar to you? Which on the list do you avoid? Are any offensive or inappropriate? What makes them so? Are there any you want to experience but have not? Are there any you want to experience more often?

Box 7.1 From Cowen and Keltner (2017)

a surge of pride, abhorrence, admiration, adoration, adrenaline rush, aesthetic appreciation, affection, aggression ...bafflement, basking, befuddlement, bewilderment, bitterness, bliss, blushing, boiling with anger, boldness... calmness, camaraderie, captivation, caring, caution, certainty, challenge, charm, cheer, cheerfulness... dark humor, daze, dedication, deep concentration, deep contemplation, deep focus, deep relief, defeat, defensiveness... eagerness, earnestness, ecstasy, ecstatic desire, edginess, egotism, elation, elevation, embarrassed relief, embarrassment... fascination, fatigue, fear, fear of missing out, fearful anger, fearful awe, fearful disgust, fearful surprise, fearlessness...giddiness, giddy anticipation, giggling, gladness, glee, gloating, gloom, glory, going ballistic, goosebumps, gratification...happiness, happy disgust, happy surprise, hate, hatred, having fun, heart sinking, heartache, heartbreak, heavenly bliss...ill temper, impatience, inadequacy, indecision, indifference, indignation, inferiority, insight, inspiration... lack of focus, laughter, lightheadedness, loathing, loneliness, longing, love, loving sympathy, low spirits, loyalty...marveling, maternal love, melancholy, mild joy, misery, mistrust, moral repugnance, mournfulness, mystification... nausea, nervous breakdown, nervous laughter, nervousness, nirvana, nonchalance, nostalgia, not feeling in control...optimism, orgasm, out-of-body experience, outrage, overexcitement...pain, panic, panic attack, paranoia, passion, patriotism, peacefulness, pensiveness, perseverance, pessimism, pity, playfulness... queasiness...rage, rapture, realization, redemption, regret, rejuvenation, relaxation, releasing tension, relief, relieved contentment... sadness, sarcasm, satiation of hunger, satiation of thirst, satisfaction, savoring, scorn, seething hatred, self-anger...tearing up laughing, tenderness, tension, terror, thankfulness, thirst, thoughtfulness, thrill, tiredness, torment...uncertainty, unease, unhappiness, unspeakable horror, urge to attack, urge to be creative, urge to escape, urge to explore... vengefulness, vigor, vindication, vitality, vulnerability...warmth, weakness, weariness, wonder, worry, wrath...yearning...zeal...

If you were to construct a 25-word list of feeling words to use with clients who may have trouble accessing or labeling emotions, which would you include? Why?

Functions of Emotions

Emotions have been theorized to operate in consistent ways. In a significant contribution (Frijda, 1988), emotions are only under one's control to a limited extent and that outside of personal control, several mechanisms account for the ways they function. The law of situational meaning refers to the rise of emotions as a response to particular meanings. The law of concern refers to emotions as a response to something that matters to the individual. The law of reality concerns the experience of emotion as tied to the perceived reality of the situation. In the law of change, emotions occur because of anticipated changes in conditions that are favorable or unfavorable. The law of habituation refers to the gradual reduction in the intensity of emotion to an event over time. The comparative feeling is the emotional experience tied to the relative meaning of an event compared to another. The final law of emotion elicitation is hedonic asymmetry. While pleasure reduces without continued conditions that produce it while pain does not reduce under continued conditions that produce it.

Identification of Emotions

Emotion must translate into something visible or auditory to be communicated. It is legitimate to wonder whether there is precision in the description that accurately captures the essence of that experience.

We assume that little goes missing in the translation of a feeling into a description, but to be more accurate, the consistency that is observed or heard is more a product of the consistency of the evidence rather than the emotional experience itself. Can we accurately name an experience of emotion with words or actions?

In a large international comparative study of facial and body expressions for emotion, 18 were reliably identified (Keltner & Cordaro, 2017). The same photos were shown in China, Japan, Korea, New Zealand, Germany, Poland, Pakistan, India, Turkey, and USA. The photos included variations in head position, gaze, and facial touching. The emotional states included amusement (head back, lips separated, jaw dropped), anger (brows furrowed, eyes wide), boredom (eyelids drooping, head tilted), confusion (eyelids narrowed, head tilted), contentment (smile, eyelids drooping), coyness (lips separated, eyes turned opposite to head turn), desire (jaw dropped, eyelids drooping), disgust (eyes rowed, nose wrinkled), embarrassment (controlled smile, head turned and down), fear (eyebrows raised and pulled together, upper eyelid raised,) happiness (Duchenne display), interest (eyebrows raised, slight smile), pain (eye tightly closed, noise wrinkled), pride (head up, eyes down), sadness (brows knitted, eyes slightly tightened), shame (head down, eyes down), surprise (eyebrows raised, upper eyelid raised, jaw dropped), and sympathy (inner eyebrow raised, lower lip raised, slightly forward) (Keltner & Cordaro, 2017).

Are there universal behavioral expressions of emotional experience? Are there emotions that do not have distinct behavioral qualities? Are some behavioral expressions open to misinterpretation? Which ones and why?

A series of experiments with varying degrees of auditory and visual cues to the emotional expression of another person found strong evidence of the value of auditory cues (Kraus, 2017). In fact, those who listened and did not observe were the most consistent in their identification of the emotions in speakers' voices. This accuracy of auditory signals of emotion is rare in studies of emotional regulation which have tended to favor visual cues. The author suggested that (a) because people have more practice using facial expression to hide their emotions, and (b) that the combined cognitive load of processing visual and auditory data together leads to less efficiency may (c) explain results that show the importance and benefit of audio over audio-visual and visual cues of emotion (Kraus, 2017).

Do you listen for emotion? What are vocal cues that you recognize as indicative of an emotional state? Do volume, speed, tone, and pitch signal emotion to you? What might they mean?

Emotions in Therapy

How do you make decisions in general—with your head or your heart? Do you "listen to your gut"? Why or why not? Do you believe that thought is more effective for decision-making than emotion? Do you believe that both processes work together? Which processes are preferred? When and why? How might you handle a difference between yourself and a client?

There has been a tendency to separate emotion from cognition and to place greater emphasis on thinking as a more consistent basis from which to make decisions (Stampley & Slaght, 2004). In psychotherapy research, it is well-established that the mood of a therapist can consciously and automatically affect information processing and judgment to impact the therapy process (Stampley & Slaght, 2004). Emotion can, however, also be considered fundamental to the humanity of the therapeutic encounter and a substantial portion of the communication and relationship upon which successful therapy takes place. Instead of attempting to isolate and control for emotion, the interaction between thought and feeling is a necessary process to consider.

Emotion is essential to learning. Neurological studies of emotion on information processing implicate the amygdala as the mediator of emotional responses and feelings (Murphy, Nimmo-Smith, & Lawrence, 2003). Processes of decision-making apparent in the frontal cortex reflect changes in response to even small changes in an emotional state (Bush, Phan, & Posner, 2000). Emotion labels experience and embed in the accounts. Memories have an emotional content that is evoked by their recollection. The somatic marker hypothesis blends emotionality with rationality to explain decision-making processes. *Because the feeling is about the body, I gave the phenomenon the technical term somatic state ("soma" is Greek for body); and because it "marks" an image, I called it a marker. Note again that I use somatic in the most general sense (that which pertains to the body) and I include both visceral and nonvisceral sensation when I refer to somatic markers* (Damasio, 1996, p. 173).

Emotional competence is the ability to be aware of the ways and extents to which different emotional experiences impact on therapy (Ciarrochi & Scott, 2006). Cognitive competence is the process of clear thinking on a complete knowledge base, and procedural competence is the acquisition and application of relevant skills (Stampley & Slaght, 2004).

Empathy

There is a great deal of neurological evidence concerning the human ability to appreciate the feelings of another. Therapists are on the front lines of this automatic experience of which they are often aware as well as unaware. This double-edged sword (Russell & Brickell, 2015) offers the opportunity to feel what another is feeling as well as the expected and unpredictable effects of an intense and uncomfortable experience. The risks inherent in constant exposure to the emotionality of clients are variable, but without therapist vulnerability to another's experience, the therapy is mechanistic and without compassion. This openness to intense emotion may be some of what draws therapists to this work. Recognition of its benefits when it is not too intense or inaccessible is evident as is its value to therapists allowing them to appreciate a client's inner experience (Najavits, 2000).

There are two primary sources of emotional impact on therapy (Stampley & Slaght, 2004). Endogenous (clinician-related) emotion refers to the preexisting conditions of the therapist before entering the therapeutic encounter. Sources may include present emotional state, temperament, as well as unconscious defenses such as unconscious anxiety, over-involvement, or emotional detachment (Stampley & Slaght, 2004). Ambient (workplace-related) emotion refers to the context of therapy and the setting within which it occurs. Sources may include work conditions amid change, interpersonal conflicts with coworkers, stress due to demands, affecting activity and motivation (Stampley & Slaght, 2004).

During interaction with a client, sources of emotion may associate with biases that are activated. For example, the fundamental attribution error explains behavior in terms of personality or conditions within which the problem occurs. Other biases include the Ego bias (self-serving distortion of probability estimates). The Chagrin Factor (anticipated regret), Outcome bias (judge decision by likely outcome), Value bias or valence effect (positively valued events are more likely to happen than negatively valued ones), and Status quo bias (alternatives that tend to perpetuate the status quo) (Stampley & Slaght, 2004).

COUNTERTRANSFERENCE

Countertransference refers to the automatic emotional reactions of the therapist toward a client that occur within and because of the therapeutic encounter (Rossberg, Karterud, Pedersen, & Friis, 2010).

> Is countertransference avoidable? Is it helpful? Should therapists attempt to neutralize it? Utilize it? How can we know when a reaction is a countertransference and when it is our own personal "stuff"? Does it matter? Why or why not?

Perceptions of another person rely on comparisons to prior experience. Emotionally laden experiences can be particularly salient and evocative (Prasko & Vyskocilova, 2010). Because of the uniqueness of every therapist and every client, every therapeutic relationship has its emotional content (Ulberg et al., 2013). Countertransference is deeply cultural. Perceptions of gender, sex, race, ethnicity, (dis)ability, age, and class are evident in assumptions, beliefs, values, and norms, of the therapist. Political and religious views are also deeply held influences (Stampley & Slaght, 2004). Preexisting views of cultural groups operate consciously and unconsciously and are evident in the therapist's conduct (Stampley & Slaght, 2004).

Views of countertransference have evolved since Freud's original conceptualization. The "narrow" view of countertransference proposed by Freud holds that the unconscious reactions of the therapist occur because of the therapists own unconscious neurotic conflicts. From this view, countertransference is problematic. The "totalistic" view, introduced in 1950 (Heiman) included all conscious and unconscious reactions to a client by the therapist (Cartwright, 2011). Countertransference is inevitable and routine. It aids in understanding the client and is an asset to the relationship (Rossberg et al., 2010). At about the same time, concepts of "subjective" and "objective" countertransference emerged (Winnicott, 1949). The objective countertransference is the therapist's realistic reaction to a client, and the subjective, based on the therapists own personal issues (Cartwright, 2011). A "moderate" definition of countertransference includes reactions that are not due to factors outside of therapy (Gelso & Carter, 1994), such as a family disagreement at home. It does include therapists' reactions that are cognitive, behavioral, affective, and sensory-based on the therapists' biases, difficulties, and conflicts, which are conscious or unconscious and triggered by the client's qualities or other aspects of the clinical encounter or relationship (Fauth, 2006). More recent definitions of countertransference suggest that therapist and client together create countertransference (Gabbard & Kay, 2001, p. 984).

Importance

Countertransference is not limited to a particular theoretical orientation (Ulberg et al., 2013). In cognitive therapy, for example, countertransference refers to automatic thoughts and emotions occurring in the therapeutic relationship that shed light onto interpersonal dynamics for clients outside of therapy (Prasko & Vyskocilova, 2010). Countertransference management appears in the American Psychological Association's Task Force on empirically supported therapy relationships as promising and probably effective (Ackerman et al., 2001). The therapeutic relationship is a significant contributor to the therapy outcome (Hill & Knox, 2009). It counts for more variance regarding immediate reactions, process, and outcomes in therapy than client characteristics or theory (Fauth, 2006). Managing the reactions of the therapist and client in the therapeutic relationship are fundamental (Gelso & Hayes, 2002; Muran, 2002; Strupp, 1980). For example, clients' self-reports of symptoms are associated with the therapist's feelings about them (Rossberg et al., 2010).

Origins

There are many potential sources of countertransference reactions (Hayes & Gelso, 2001). Two of the most prominent theories of countertransference origins are developmental and cultural. From a developmental perspective, prior life experience and experiences lead to reactions to others that are, to some extent, projected. Relationships and experiences with significant people, such as parents, siblings, teachers, and neighbors, are typically the origins (Prasko & Vyskocilova, 2010). Instead of viewing early traumatic life experiences, this view incorporates all early life relationships that were in any way inconsistent with expectations or produced conflict. Because it is unusual to find anyone whose needs were met perfectly during childhood, there is potential for all to have developmentally rooted countertransference reactions (Prasko & Vyskocilova, 2010).

Culture "includes all the rules and regulations that govern a way of life, both conscious (formally stated beliefs and feelings) and unconscious (informal or implicit beliefs and feelings)" (Stampley & Slaight, 2004). The cultural background, personal and socialization experiences contribute to a sense of self and others. Values, theories, as well as biases and prejudices all play a role in countertransference and affect the therapy provided to different clients (Stampey & Slaight, 2004). Worldviews, attitudes about different groups, politics, religion, and morality all influence countertransference (Lane, 1986). These may be rooted in beliefs, social and environmental influences, and personal life experiences (Stampley & Slaight, 2004).

Family beliefs and messages can include a range of issues. The issues often include expectations about support and roles. To what extent are family members responsible for other family members? Who takes on that role and why or why not?

Knowledge and perceptions of social history such as slavery, the Holocaust, internment camps, Residential Schools, the 60's Scoop, and migration play a role in reactions to present-day events. The media plays a significant role in views and expectations of self and others. Less popular and often more extreme views are evident in alternative media locations (Stampley & Slaight, 2004). Personal life experiences with clients as well as others who "confirm" beliefs and expectations about individuals that are in some way similar to each other also have a profound influence. These can be positive or negative experiences, acceptable or unacceptable judgments, with low or high expectations as a result (Stampley & Slaight, 2004).

As a therapist, are there, clients, because of injustice, you have strong feelings for? Which groups and why? What are the feelings? Guilt, anger, sadness, fear? What do those feelings tell you about how you would greet and interact with the client? Would you be aware of your reaction to your sense of injustice? How would you recognize it as yours and not your client's?

Research

There are two main sets of considerations for studies that examine countertransference. These include the perspective and the stimuli. The perspectives include the therapists themselves, observers, as well as supervisors. The stimuli include video and live encounters.

Studies focusing on the therapists' experiences focus on the emotional state during sessions. There is an assumption that therapists can and will report their emotions. Existing research has found that therapists, despite some of their experience located in the unconscious, can reliably identify different countertransference emotions (Brody & Farber, 1996; Imhof, 1991). Also, therapists, despite the potential to report only socially acceptable emotions, do not report only those that put them in a favorable light (Najavits, 2000). Observers who are trained to identify and rate therapists' emotions have the advantage of minimizing social desirability, but the disadvantage of being only able to infer the therapists' emotions (Colli & Ferri, 2015). While the supervisor has some insight into the therapist's expression of emotional reaction and more reliably infer it than a non-familiar observer, the relationship between therapist and supervisor may impact the quality of ratings (Colli & Ferri, 2015).

The use of live sessions or predetermined vignettes has trade-offs. In the case of live sessions, they have strong external validity and applicability to actual work with clients but may have limits on the consistency of degree and type of prompts made for therapist reactions. Likewise, taped vignettes have consistency in degree and type of stimulus, but less direct applicability to typical daily practice (Colli & Ferri, 2015). Both prerecorded and live exposure can utilize systems for organizing therapists' emotional reactions. For example, the QUAINT method (Connolly et al., 1996) includes judges' ratings of relationships as described by clients and issues in their narratives within sessions.

> Which of the ways that research accesses countertransference reactions would be useful for you to use in your practice? Why? Which would be less effective? Why?

Reactions to Clients

Feeling words have been used to describe therapists' reactions to clients. Variations of checklists of words exist for (a) therapists from different theoretical orientations, who rated their reactions to (b) adult and adolescent clients in (c) inpatient and outpatient settings, for (d) mental health assessment and treatment, at the (e) beginning and end of treatment. These feeling word checklists have an underlying factor structure. They range in number as well as the type of factor (i.e. unipolar or bipolar).

In 1982 the professional styles of nurses and other staff members, as well as responses to different diagnoses and particular patients were explored with feeling words (Whyte, Constantopoulos, & Bevans, 1982). A 30-word checklist yielded seven bipolar factors (Holmqvist & Armelius, 1994), and then a 48-word version with four unipolar factors (Holmqvist, 2001). The most recent version includes 30 feelings. The words are: Affectionate, Aloof, Anxious, Attentive, Bored, Calm, Cautious, Clever, Confident, Disliked, Distressed, Dominate, Embarrassed, Enthusiastic, Happy, Helpful, Helpless, Important, Inadequate, Indifferent, Insecure, Motherly, Objective. Overwhelmed, Receptive, Rejected, Sleepy, Stupid, Threatened, Tired of, and Total control (Dahl, Røssberg, Bøgwald, Gabbard, & Høglend, 2012).

Underlying factors exist for different sets of feeling words. A four-factor solution included "Therapist in Conflict with Self" (e.g. confused, doubting one's competence), "Therapist Focused on Own Needs" (e.g. insufficiently paid, bored), "Positive Connection" (e.g. enjoyment, liking, empathy), and "Therapist in Conflict with the Patient" (e.g. power struggles, feeling manipulated by the patient) (Najavits, 2000). Another four-factor solution yielded Confident, Inadequate, Disengaged, and Neutral (Ulberg et al., 2013). An eight-factor solution found (1) Helpful vs. Unhelpful; (2) Accepting vs. Rejecting; (3) Close vs. Distant; (4) Autonomy vs. Controlled (de Vogel & de Ruiter, 2004). Another eight-factor solution yielded: (1) Overwhelmed/Disorganized, (2) Helpless/Inadequate, (3) Positive, (4) Special/Overinvolved, (5) Sexualized, (6) Disengaged, (7) Parental/Protective, and (8) Criticized/Mistreated (Prasko et al., 2010).

Therapists' Emotions

Following identification of underlying factor structure among therapists' emotional reactions to clients, research has been done to measure the extent to which they covary with client issues and treatment outcomes. Therapists emotional reactions have been linked to types of countertransference. These include feelings of admiration, fascination (admiring countertransference), fear, insecurity (overprotective), fascination, "trance" (erotic), fear, anxiety, shame (apprehensive), anger, resonance (aggressive), apprehension (distrustful), and contempt (derogatory) (Prasko et al., 2010).

Client characteristics are a source of variation in therapists' emotional responses. More intense client emotions are associated with more intense therapist emotions (Imhof, 1991; Najavits, 2000). Clients' diagnoses contribute to therapists' emotional variation. For example, therapist anger occurs with client personality disorders, protectiveness with suicidal depression, and hopelessness with psychosis (Najavits, 2000). Client behaviors such as aggression, withdrawal, and suicidality associate with therapist anger and helplessness (Rossberg, Karterud, Pedersen, & Friis, 2008). More considerable client distress associated with more positive therapist emotion at the start of therapy, but more negative emotion at the end of therapy (Rossberg et al., 2008).

Many of us have a particular sensitivity to and meaning associated with specific emotions. One of the more challenging for many of us is anger. How do you respond to anger in another? What if that individual is angry at someone or something other than you? What if that individual is angry at you? What do you tell yourself or take it to mean when you conclude that another person is angry with you? How has it or would it play out with you as the therapist of a client who is angry with you?

Different therapists also have different types of emotional responses. More experienced therapists tend to be more comfortable with their emotional reactions in therapy than early-career therapists (Connoly et al., 1996). Male therapists report more sexual attraction to clients than female therapists (Pope & Tabachnick, 1993). Therapists' feelings of importance and confidence are higher for patients with lower symptomatology, and more likely to be bored, overwhelmed with higher symptomatology (Rossberg et al., 2010). Theoretical orientation does not appear to contribute predictably to client reactions by therapists (Colli & Ferri, 2015).

Therapy characteristics are related to therapists' emotional reactions. More anger in the therapist's voice during the initial interview, the lower follow up by clients with substance abuse treatment (Milmoe, Rosenthal, Blane, Chafetz, & Wolf, 1967). Clients who are liked by their therapists are more likely to be viewed in situational terms, while clients whom therapists do not like are more likely to be seen in dispositional terms (Stampley & Slaght, 2004). The more positive the emotional reactions of the therapist to a client, the more likely is symptom change (Rossberg et al., 2010). Therapists who felt rejected and inadequate were related to the client's lack of improvement or deterioration (Rossberg et al., 2008).

How do you know how you are coming across to a client? What do you recognize in yourself? Are there behaviors or thoughts? Which emotions show up when you are uncomfortable and comfortable with a client?

Triggers and Manifestations

Triggers refer to aspects of the therapy encounter that stir emotion. These vary considerably from therapists to therapist. Several areas exist. Client characteristics such as physical appearance and cultural group membership, or reminder of a significant person in the therapist's life (Hayes & Gelso, 2001). Therapy content touching on a therapist's unresolved conflict can be triggering, such as family issues and death, as well as sexuality, health, and religious or spiritual concerns (Stampley & Spaight, 2004). The process concerns how the therapist and client speak to one another. Triggers in this area include who dominates, emotional expression, premature endings, within sessions as well as between or across sessions (Hayes & Gelso, 2001).

Manifestations are behavioral, affective, and cognitive. Behaviors may be avoidance or compensation (Rosenberger & Hayes, 2002; Stampley & Spaight, 2004). While anxiety has been the most often studied, affect reaction, anger, sadness, boredom is also often noted (Stampley & Spaight, 2004). Because anxiety is a consistently triggered reaction, therapists who have higher trait anxiety are more likely to experience more countertransference (Hayes & Gelso, 2001). Cognitive manifestations often include some level of distortion. Reactions may exaggerate or underrecognize certain aspects of the client's experience, overstate or understate the amount of time devoted to the topics. The more therapists perceive clients to be like themselves, the more they liked them and were less likely to view clients are overly unlike themselves (Hayes & Gelso, 2001).

If a client reminds you of yourself are you likely to feel more comfortable with that client? More effective with that client? Why is feeling comfortable and effective based on similarity a benefit, and why may it also be a challenge? What about a difference. If a client strikes you as very different from yourself, how do you react? How can that be helpful or unhelpful to a client?

Recognizing Countertransference

Some issues that may arise include looking forward to a session with a particular client, worried about it or possibly dreading it; strong feelings toward a client—either supportive or unsupportive; letting a "good session" extend past the time limit, making accommodations in your schedule for a client to be seen earlier or later; looking forward to or fearful of termination (Prasko et al., 2010). It can be helpful to consider the reaction one is having toward a client, whether it is too big for the situation, what is bothersome about the client, what one would like to or not like to discuss with them. It can be helpful also to consider what one may have missed because of the strong reaction.

Summary

- There has been a tendency to separate emotion from cognition and to place greater emphasis on thinking as a more consistent and sounder basis from which to operate in counseling and psychotherapy.
- There is ample neurological evidence of the human ability to appreciate the feelings of another. Therapists are on the front lines of this automatic experience, of which they are often mostly aware as well as unaware.
- Countertransference is the automatic emotional reactions of the therapist toward client that occur within and are a result of the clinical encounter. From a developmental perspective, previous life experience and painful experiences lead to reactions to others that are, to some extent, projected.
- The cultural background, personal and socialization experiences contribute to a sense of self and others. Values, theories, as well as biases and prejudices all play a role in countertransference and impact the therapy provided.

Discussion Questions

1. Is therapist empathy necessary for client change? Why or why not?
2. How do your facial expressions change in response to emotional state? Practice in front of a mirror—your happy, sad, angry, contemptuous, and suspicious reactions. Practice in dyads with a partner. What does your partner notice that you do not? Practice with someone who knows you well. What does that person notice in you and you do not?
3. Think of the last time you encountered a stranger who reminded you of someone you know. What did you feel when you noticed

them? What was it about that stranger that reminded you of the person? What does your reaction tell you about your relationship with that person? What does your reaction tell you about that stranger? Fit your responses into the following categories: origins, triggers, manifestations, management, and effects (Fauth, 2006).

REFERENCES

Ackerman, S. J., Benjamin, L. S., Beutler, L. E., Gelso, C. J., Goldfried, M. R., Hill, C., … & Rainer, J. (2001). Empirically supported therapy relationships: Conclusions and recommendations of the Division 29 Task Force. *Psychotherapy: Theory, Research, Practice, Training, 38*(4), 495.

Barrett, L. F., Lewis, M., & Haviland-Jones, J. M. (Eds.). (2016). *Handbook of emotions.* New York: Guilford.

Brody, E. M., & Farber, B. A. (1996). The effects of therapist experience and patient diagnosis on countertransference. *Psychotherapy: Theory, Research, Practice, Training, 33*(3), 372.

Bush, G., Luu, P., & Posner, M. I. (2000). Cognitive and emotional influences in anterior cingulate cortex. *Trends in Cognitive Sciences, 4*(6), 215–222.

Cartwright, C. (2011). Transference, countertransference, and reflective practice in cognitive therapy. *Clinical Psychologist, 15*(3), 112–120.

Ciarrochi, J., & Scott, G. (2006). The link between emotional competence and well-being: A longitudinal study. *British Journal of Guidance and Counselling, 34*(2), 231–243.

Colli, A., & Ferri, M. (2015). Patient personality and therapist countertransference. *Current Opinion in Psychiatry, 28*(1), 46–56.

Connolly, M. B., Crits-Christoph, P., Demorest, A., Azarian, K., Muenz, L., & Chittams, J. (1996). Varieties of transference patterns in psychotherapy. *Journal of Consulting and Clinical Psychology, 64*(6), 1213.

Cowen, A. S., & Keltner, D. (2017). Self-report captures 27 distinct categories of emotion bridged by continuous gradients. *Proceedings of the National Academy of Sciences, 114*(38), E7900–E7909.

Dahl, H. S. J., Røssberg, J. I., Bøgwald, K. P., Gabbard, G. O., & Høglend, P. A. (2012). Countertransference feelings in one year of individual therapy: An evaluation of the factor structure in the Feeling Word Checklist-58. *Psychotherapy Research, 22*(1), 12–25.

Damasio, A. R. (1996). The somatic marker hypothesis and the possible functions of the prefrontal cortex. Philosophical Transactions of the Royal Society of London. *Series B: Biological Sciences, 351*(1346), 1413–1420.

Demoulin, S., Leyens, J. P., Paladino, M. P., Rodriguez-Torres, R., Rodriguez-Perez, A., & Dovidio, J. (2004). Dimensions of "uniquely" and "non-uniquely" human emotions. *Cognition and Emotion, 18*(1), 71–96.

de Vogel, V., & de Ruiter, C. (2004). Differences between clinicians and researchers in assessing risk of violence in forensic psychiatric patients. *Journal of Forensic Psychiatry & Psychology, 15*(1), 145–164.

Fauth, J. (2006). Toward more (and better) countertransference research. *Psychotherapy: Theory, Research, Practice, Training, 43*(1), 16–31.

Frijda, N. H. (1988). The laws of emotion. *American Psychologist, 43*(5), 349.

Gabbard, G. O., & Kay, J. (2001). The fate of integrated treatment: Whatever happened to the biopsychosocial psychiatrist? *American Journal of Psychiatry, 158*(12), 1956–1963.

Gelso, C. J., & Carter, J. A. (1994). Components of the psychotherapy relationship: Their interaction and unfolding during treatment. *Journal of Counseling Psychology, 41*(3), 296.

Gelso, C. J., & Hayes, J. A. (2002). The management of countertransference. In J. C. Norcross (Ed.), *Psychotherapy relationships that work: Therapist contributions and responsiveness to patients* (pp. 267–283). New York, NY: Oxford University Press.

Hayes, J. A., & Gelso, C. J. (2001). Clinical implications of research on countertransference: Science informing practice. *Journal of Clinical Psychology, 57*(8), 1041–1051.

Hill, C. E., & Knox, S. (2009). Processing the therapeutic relationship. *Psychotherapy Research, 19*(1), 13–29.

Holmqvist, R. (2001). Patterns of consistency and deviation in therapists' countertransference feelings. *Journal of Psychotherapy Practice & Research, 10*(2), 104–116.

Holmqvist, R., & Armelius, B. Å. (1994). Emotional reactions to psychiatric patients: Analysis of a feeling checklist. *Acta Psychiatrica Scandinavica, 90*(3), 204–209.

Horton, R. (2006). *Refining theory and practice in the cultural psychology of emotion: Tibetan "anger" and the roots of the modern Tibetan commitment to nonviolence* (Unpublished doctoral dissertation), University of Chicago.

Imhof, J. E. (1991). Countertransference issues in alcoholism and drug addiction. *Psychiatric Annals, 21*(5), 292–306.

Joseph, C. (2001). *The virtues as a cultural domain: A study of Arabic Speaking Muslims* (Unpublished doctoral dissertation), University of Chicago.

Keltner, D., & Cordaro, D. T. (2017). Understanding multimodal emotional expressions: Recent advances in basic emotion theory. In Jose-Miguel Fernandez-Dols & James Russell (Eds.), *The science of facial expression* (pp. 57–76). London: Oxford University Press.

Kohler, C. G., Turner, T., Stolar, N. M., Bilker, W. B., Brensinger, C. M., Gur, R. E., et al. (2004). Differences in facial expressions of four universal emotions. *Psychiatry Research, 128*(3), 235–244.

Kraus, M. W. (2017). Voice-only communication enhances empathic accuracy. *American Psychologist, 72*(7), 644.

Lane, F. M. (1986). Transference and countertransference: Definitions of terms. In H. Meyers (ED.), *Between analyst and patient: New dimensions in countertransference and transference* (pp. 237–256). London, UK: Routledge.

Milmoe, S., Rosenthal, R., Blane, H. T., Chafetz, M. E., & Wolf, I. (1967). The doctor's voice: Postdictor of successful referral of alcoholic patients. *Journal of Abnormal Psychology, 72*(1), 78.

Muran, J. C. (2002). A relational approach to understanding change: Plurality and contextualism in a psychotherapy research program. *Psychotherapy Research, 12*(2), 113–138.

Murphy, F. C., Nimmo-Smith, I. A. N., & Lawrence, A. D. (2003). Functional neuroanatomy of emotions: A meta-analysis. *Cognitive, Affective, & Behavioral Neuroscience, 3*(3), 207–233.

Najavits, L. M. (2000). Researching therapist emotions and countertransference. *Cognitive and Behavioral Practice, 7*(3), 322–328.

Plutchik, R. (1997). The circumplex as a general model of the structure of emotions and personality. In R. Plutchik & H. R. Conte (Eds.), *Circumplex models of personality and emotions* (pp. 17–45). Washington, DC: American Psychological Association.

Pope, K. S., & Tabachnick, B. G. (1993). Therapists' anger, hate, fear, and sexual feelings: National survey of therapist responses, client characteristics, critical events, formal complaints, and training. *Professional Psychology: Research and Practice, 24*(2), 142.

Prasko, J., & Vyskocilova, J. (2010). Countertransference during supervision in cognitive behavioral therapy. *Activitas Nervosa Superior Rediviva, 52*(4), 253–262.

Prasko, J., Diveky, T., Grambal, A., Kamaradova, D., Mozny, P., Sigmundova, Z., ... & Vyskocilova, J. (2010). Transference and countertransference in cognitive behavioral therapy. *Biomedical Papers, 154*(3), 189–198.

Rosenberger, E. W., & Hayes, J. A. (2002). Origins, consequences, and management of countertransference: A case study. *Journal of Counseling Psychology, 49*(2), 221.

Rossberg, J. I., Karterud, S., Pedersen, G., & Friis, S. (2008). Specific personality traits evoke different countertransference reactions: An empirical study. *The Journal of Nervous and Mental Disease, 196*(9), 702–708.

Rossberg, J. I., Karterud, S., Pedersen, G., & Friis, S. (2010). Psychiatric symptoms and countertransference feelings: An empirical investigation. *Psychiatry Research, 178*(1), 191–195.

Russell, M., & Brickell, M. (2015). The "double-edge sword" of human empathy: A unifying neurobehavioral theory of compassion stress injury. *Social Sciences, 4*(4), 1087–1117.

Sherif, M. A. (1975). *Ghazali's theory of virtue*. Albany, NY: SUNY Press.

Shweder, R. A., Haidt, J., Horton, R., & Joseph, C. (2008). The cultural psychology of the emotions: Ancient and renewed. In M. Lewis, J. M. Haviland-Jones, & L. F. Barrett (Eds.), *Handbook of emotions* (pp. 409–427). New York, NY: The Guilford Press.

Stampley, C., & Slaght, E. (2004). Cultural countertransference as a clinical obstacle. *Smith College Studies in Social Work, 74*(2), 333–347.

Strupp, H. H. (1980). Success and failure in time-limited psychotherapy: A systematic comparison of two cases: Comparison 1. *Archives of General Psychiatry, 37*(5), 595–603.

Thoits, P. A. (1989). The sociology of emotions. *Annual Review of Sociology, 15*(1), 317–342.

Ulberg, R., Falkenberg, A. A., Nerdal, T. B., Johannessen, H., Olsen, J. E., Eide, T. K., et al. (2013). Countertransference feelings when treating teenagers: A psychometric evaluation of the Feeling Word Checklist–24. *American Journal of Psychotherapy, 67*(4), 347–358.

Whyte, C. R., Constantopoulos, C., & Bevans, H. G. (1982). Types of countertransference identified by Q- analysis. *British Journal of Medical Psychology, 55*(2), 187–201.

Winnicott, D. W. (1949). Hate in the counter-transference. *International Journal of Psycho-Analysis, 30*, 69–74.

CHAPTER 8

Woundedness and Boundaries

WOUNDED HEALER

The wounded healer is a concept central to the relationship and therapy process. It refers to the connection that woundedness for the therapist and client each separately have experienced. The therapist, having progressed along with their healing, is positioned to assist a client to explore and heal. It is a process of compassion that flows from the therapist to the client and then back to the therapist (Stone, 2008).

> What have you heard before about the concept of the wounded healer? How do you envision the role of the therapist in terms of their illness and healing? Is it necessary for you as a therapist to have had a similar experience to a client to be helpful to that client? Is it necessary to have had personal struggles and to have resolved them to be helpful? Can your wounds get in the way of helping a client?

The wounded healer has origins in Greek mythology (Kirmayer, 2003). Asklepios, the son of the god Apollo and the mortal Koronis, was wounded before birth by an arrow from Apollo's sister Artemis. At birth, he was given to the healer Chirton, a centaur. Chirton himself suffered from an accidental and incurable wound. Living a life of chronic pain

© The Author(s) 2019
J. D. Brown, *Reflective Practice of Counseling and Psychotherapy in a Diverse Society*, https://doi.org/10.1007/978-3-030-24505-4_8

and suffering, he was unable to heal himself, but he could heal and teach others (Conti-O'Hare, 1998). It was his foster father Chirton who taught Askepios the "art of healing" with "the capacity to be at home in the darkness of suffering and there to find seeds of light and recovery" (Stone, 2008).

Woundedness and the power to heal are very closely associated. The healer's exposure to diseases provides unique insight regarding the significance of the affliction. As one chosen for exposure to disease and healing through supernatural forces, the healer's survival also provides the knowledge of both illness as well as the power to heal (Kirmayer, 2003). Essential aspects of this are that (a) the healer must be vulnerable, and (b) only the affliction, not the person, can be healed (Kirmayer, 2003).

The Wounded Healer Archetype

Archetypes are qualities of experience thought to be universal (Kirmayer, 2003). They appear as ideas, images or dreams that the therapist or client have as part of their experience (Conti-O'Hare, 1998). The archetype signifies a likelihood that a client's inner healer will become stronger through the therapists self-woundedness and openness (Conti-O'Hare, 1998). This archetype is stirred in the therapist by the client's wounds activating the therapists own inner healer (Sedgwick, 1994). Once the therapists' wounds are activated, their healing process provides power to assist the client with understanding and change (Zerubavel & Wright, 2012).

Carl Jung first referenced the wounded healer archetype. His views changed significantly over the course of his career from early notes about the need for therapists to be free from their own personal struggles in order to keep their hands clean, to his later writings where he noted that "only the wounded physician heals" (Jung & Jung, 1963, p. 134). In contrast to Freud, Jung supported the use of countertransference as a means by which the patient could be understood (Jung, 1951). The countertransference he described was an unconscious transfer of the disease from the patient to the therapist (Laskowski & Pellicore, 2002). The therapist "quite literally takes over the sufferings of his patient and shares them with him" (Laskowski & Pellicore, 2002). Both therapist and client are "altered" or "transformed" through the dialectical healing process (Laskowski & Pellicore, 2002).

Which of these views resonates most strongly with you as a therapist? Is it accurate that only the wounded therapist can help clients? Is it more useful to keep your "hands clean"? Is it possible to live without becoming wounded at some point? Are there wounds from which it is necessary to take a break from practicing? In what ways can your wounds and healing help in your work with clients? How can they get in the way?

Denial of the Therapists' Wounds

Separation of the therapist's and client's wounds and healing are necessary in many Western approaches to counseling and psychotherapy. However, the wounded healer archetype suggests that denial of the healer within the client and woundedness in the therapist serve to create and sustain pathology as well as passivity (Laskowski & Pellicore, 2002). Not only is a therapist's woundedness an opening for both client and therapist, but also an opportunity for the client to offer some help to the therapist. Searles (1975) in (Kirmayer, 2003) "found over and over that stalemates in treatment, when explored sufficiently, involve the analyst's receiving a kind of therapeutic support from the patient of which both patient and analyst have been unconscious." Without any acknowledgment of their woundedness, the therapist may promote a splitting from the client, pitting the healthy against the unhealthy, with the healthy side fostering dependency in the unhealthy (Zerubavel & Wright, 2012).

Embrace of the Therapists' Wounds

"I have come to appreciate the fact that patients will have an impact on me. Indeed, an absence of impact may mean as much as its presence" (Sedgwick, 2016). However, this openness to the client, while essential to their own ability to be helpful and authoritative, may also come at a cost to the therapist (Laskowski & Pellicore, 2002). In order to be effective, therapists must be making progress on their healing and be further along that path than their clients (Zerubavel & Wright, 2012). It is the stigma of woundedness that may prevent some therapists from acknowledging their limits and pressing on to prove that they are, indeed, healthy or healed (Zerubavel & Wright, 2012).

Consider what wounds you carry and how much progress you have made in your healing. What have you learned about yourself? About healing yourself? About healing another? Is there more work for you to do concerning your healing? If so, what will you do to ensure that you keep making progress?

Across cultural differences, the woundedness can provide a commonality of experience. Kirmayer notes that "in intercultural encounters, clinicians are often in a state of vulnerability, confusion, and powerlessness. They may feel inadequate, incompetent and dull, and be vicariously traumatized by patients' stories of suffering. The ability to deal with these threats to the self, and (re)wounding, without retaliation or appropriation of the healing function, depends on integrating the notion of the wounded-healer" (Kirmayer, 2003).

Development of the Wounded Healer

The "doctor knows, even unconsciously, that he did not choose this profession by chance and must come to terms with why he chose that profession" (Groesbeck, 1975, p. 135). Through the perspective of the archetype, the therapist has chosen a path to heal woundedness in others because of the woundedness they have suffered (Conti-O'Hare, 1998). Hanshew (1998) cites Goldberg in "those drawn to psychotherapy are impelled by the instinctual disposition … of a psyche whose vulnerability has never fully healed" and in the necessity of personal struggle as a requirement for growth as a therapist and as a resource for clients.

A model of development for a therapist's inner healer begins with an acknowledgment of their woundedness. This acknowledgment may be the most challenging step to take, particularly early in a career where one is acutely aware of the gatekeeping function supervisors have and the importance of their recommendations for entry into the profession. Following acknowledgment, the development includes sufficient healing of oneself to the point of recognition that the experiences are characteristic of one who is both vulnerable and strong.

The discovery of this potential offers a new appreciation for life. A strengthening of meaning and purpose follows it, and with it, the ability to connect interpersonally and empathetically (Zerubavel & Wright, 2012). With each new encounter and client, the therapist is required to return to an evolving and changing sense of self that touches their wounding. "We could say, without too much exaggeration, that a good half of every treatment that probes at all deeply consists in the doctor's examining himself, for only what he can put right in himself can he hope to put right in the patient" (Kirmayer, 2003).

Consider your own prior experience as a therapist or client. How might you tell whether the healer is the inner healer of the client or the therapist's healing potential? Does this distinction matter? Why or why not?

Healing in the Therapeutic Encounter

The archetype of the wounded healer may be a helpful lens through which to view the relationship, therapeutic encounter, healing process as well as roles of therapist and client. The potential for fostering empathy and hope are desirable effects. However, while the archetype encourages therapist vulnerability, it does not speak as powerfully to safety. Therapist's awareness of their recovery from woundedness as well as recognition that their healing path is unique to themselves is essential. Recovery is not a linear process. Shifts, setbacks, as well as periods of stagnation, occur in addition to growth (Zerubavel & Wright, 2012). Careful and honest monitoring of self by self and trusted others through supervision is a means by which to remain cognizant of the therapist's process. Different periods during a therapist's recovery affect their vulnerabilities and intersect with clients' experiences of their wounds and healing. Therapists connect powerfully with clients. However, the connection can also lead to intentional as well as unanticipated overextensions. Therapists live with a paradox that caring is proper, but too much caring or overinvolvement can harm themselves (Montgomery, 1991; Stone, 2008).

How do you feel about the concept of healing? What is the relationship between healing and therapy? How are they similar and different from each other? To what extent does good therapy include healing?

BOUNDARIES

Boundaries are ways of relating to clients such as through the roles of client and therapist (Owen, 1997). They may be formalized guidelines that are requirements and clearly state minimum standards of acceptability (Owen, 1997). Boundaries concern the regulations that therapists are to comply with and clarity for clients about who will do what when as well as what would be out of bounds (Barnett, 2015; Knapp & Slattery, 2004; Pietkiewicz & Skowrońska-Włoch, 2017). They have a significant effect on the process and outcome in therapy.

Boundaries offer containment for both therapist and client. They keep the focus on what the client is bringing to the encounter (Bridges, 1999). Boundaries may be psychological or physical (Hay, 2018). They provide "A therapeutic frame which defines a set of roles for the participants in the therapeutic process'...and provide a foundation for this relationship by fostering a sense of safety and the belief that the clinician will always act in the client's best interest" (Barnett, 2015; Smith & Fitzpatrick, 1995, p. 500). They are personal, sexual, family, ethnic, provincial, social class, and cultural (Hay, 2018). In this nested model, it follows that any change in one boundary has effects on the other boundaries.

There is also a moral sense to boundaries as good and bad or right and wrong (Owen, 1997). Boundaries have edges that define what is appropriate and inappropriate helping behaviors are (Austin, Bergum, Nuttgens, & Peternelj-Taylor, 2006). The edges define what is acceptable and unacceptable (Heru, Strong, Price, & Recupero, 2006). They distinguish between a therapeutic relationship and a friendship or a friendly relationship (Austin et al., 2006).

Boundaries reflect influence and control (Austin et al., 2006). They may be negotiated to an extent for the protection of the therapist and client (Pietkiewicz & Skowrońska-Włoch, 2017). For clients, they offer safety psychologically to express themselves (Westergaard, 2013). They protect clients from the therapist's position and expertise, and the personal nature of information shared by the client disproportionately with the therapist (Gabbard, 1996). Clients may "gain a clearer sense of ourselves and our relationship to others" (Hermansson, 1997, p. 5). Boundaries also help therapists by giving them psychological space within which to operate (Dorpat, 1977; Owen, 1997).

One major area of discussion is the boundaries in online relationships with clients. How do you use technology to communicate with clients? What are the advantages and disadvantages? Are there ways that a current or potential client could access your online activity? How so? What are the pros and cons of this?

Gray Areas

There are many boundaries, and they are always in play. They may include theories, phases, cultures, individual/family/systemic, third parties, and information sharing (Hermansson, 1997). Therapists must be sensitive to read client cues that indicate their perceived position and comfort or discomfort relative to the boundaries (Laungani, 2004). If boundaries are too strict, they constrain and dehumanize (Hermansson, 1997). They can also be thick or thin, and while permeability allows for an authentic connection for sharing feelings while providing some containment for them, limits must also exist (Bridges, 1999). It is part of the challenge presented by clients at times to help them stretch their boundaries (Hermansson, 1997).

Types of Boundaries

The pressure for clarity in boundaries comes from risk management and treatment control (Hermansson, 1997). Boundary crossing may be very helpful but, with potential for abuse (Hermansson, 1997). Instead of either-or definitions, it is possible to consider boundaries as permeable and flexible (Pugh, 2006). While boundaries are good places to start with therapy—whom what when, where and how—there will be more pressing issues to which an immediate response is warranted (Owen, 1997).

A variety of boundaries have been described (Hartmann, 1997). These include perceptual boundaries (between sensory inputs, sensory focus or "bandwidth," around perceptual entities), thoughts and feelings (between two thoughts or two feelings, between thought and feeling), around thoughts and feelings (free association), states of awareness or states of consciousness (sleep-dream-wake boundaries, between sleep and waking, between dreaming and waking, in and around the dream, daydreaming), those related to play, related to memory (early memories, recent memories and memory organization, personal past, future plans) as well as around oneself (body boundaries), barrier against stimuli, the skin as a boundary, posture and musculature as boundaries, personal space, interpersonal boundaries between conscious and unconscious and between id, ego, and superego (defense mechanisms as boundaries), and identity (sexual identity, age identity: between adult and child, constancy of identity, group boundaries).

> For each of the following, what are your personal comfort zones? How might those be similar and different for clients? How would you know? In what ways could a client's perception of what is permissible override your comfort? (1) personal space, (2) locations for sessions, (3) timing and duration of sessions, (4) emergency out of office contact

Cultural Considerations

While we have cross-cultural encounters in therapy, frequently these differences are unexplored. Migration and electronic communication bring people closer together than ever before, but often around dominant worldviews with assumptions that we do not examine. It is naive to think that all peoples are Westernized (Bojuwoye, 2001). "The fact is that culture is not something that can easily be wished away or wiped out completely as its legacies continue to remain in the people. Ideas and rules that direct people's behaviours, the form of things people hold in their minds, and their modes of perceiving, relating and otherwise interpreting do not just die out entirely but continue to exist within the existential and general milieu of the people" (Bojuwoye, 2001). For example, Shamanism has a basis in spiritual energy and transformation with help from, or dependent on, divine entities. In contrast, Western talk therapy has tended to focus on the agency of the individual and control over forces within (Austin et al., 2006).

What role does spirituality play in therapy? Is it a commanding presence on sickness and wellness? Are there times when a problem is more spiritual than psychological? How would you know? What would you do? Should indigenous healing be integrated into therapy?

Knowing one's view of therapy and the roles of therapist and client is essential. For example, there may be very different understandings of what is supposed to happen and why it is supposed to happen in therapy. A client might assume a vertical model where the therapist is an expert, and the client is seeking direct advice and guidance. However, therapists are often trained to take an egalitarian stance, within which the therapist does not provide direct assistance but guides a client to the discovery of their answers (Laungani, 2004). From the latter perceptive, the assumption is that the individual has control, the context is neutral, destiny and divine intervention have small if any role in personal change. In this case, the therapist is operating from a perspective which is assumed to be accurate, but is, in fact, culturally embedded and assumed to be true for all (Laungani, 2004).

How might you handle such differences in expectation? If a client wants direction and you encourage exploration, are you helping or hindering their process? If a client wants direct answers and you keep asking questions, are you being disrespectful or insensitive? In such cases, should the therapist become more directive? When is the context of the problem? Should a therapist challenge a client's beliefs in destiny or spiritual intervention? Is it possible to do so in a respectful way?

Crossings, Slopes, and Violations

Crossing a boundary is "a departure from a commonly accepted practice that may or may not benefit the client" (Smith & Fitzpatrick, 1995, p. 501) while a violation is a behavior that is known to be harmful to a client (Audet, 2011; Gutheil & Gabbard, 1998). A crossing can be justified clinically, concerning a particular theory or activity, specific need or exceptional circumstance, while a violation is because of an exceptional need of the therapist (Barnett, 2015).

Consider the following boundaries and the extent to which you consider them to be helpful and harmful? (a) Telling a client about the date you went on the evening prior. (b) Buying groceries at a client's partner's store. (c) Meeting a client in a public location. (d) Hiring the son of a client to file paperwork because he wants to learn how to become a therapist. (e) Accepting artwork from a client who is an artist (Austin et al., 2006).

Crossing a boundary has both potential benefits and drawbacks. It is difficult to know when it is and is not appropriate. Strict limits are clear but potentially limiting to the client, while flexible limits/guidelines are vague but potentially helpful to the client (Hermansson, 1997). A crossing with significant benefit is the connection it permits emotional closeness and entry into the client's "life space," which essential for the development of empathy (Hermansson, 1997). A strict and distant relationship, while maintaining impeccable boundaries, may detract from the alliance (Hermansson, 1997).

Are boundary crossings a precursor to boundary violations (Gabbard, 1996). Does a boundary crossing open the door for a violation? Why or why not?

Self-Disclosure

Self-disclosure is acceptable within most schools of thought in counseling and psychotherapy. While psychoanalytic practice in its classical form necessitates a distance between therapist and client, relational practice would treat relational closeness and sense of humanity as fundamental for providing feedback and beneficial experience. Humanist practice is similarly highly disclosing to show authenticity and fallibility of the therapist (and all of humankind) as a product of the human condition. Feminist practice also includes closeness, connection, and disclosure to clarify the sense of self as part of a group within a political context. Cognitive-behavioral practice also utilizes disclosure as a means by which to normalize an experience (Knox & Hill, 2003). Such theoretical differences can, however, in therapy practice, go to an extreme. For example, a humanist therapist who remains silent to encourage a client toward self-expression may leave a client imagining and worrying (Dindia & Allen, 1992).

> How much are you drawn to self-disclose in therapy? When do you do it? Why do you do it? What is the difference between helpful and unhelpful self-disclosure? How do you know?

Self-disclosure has been found through research to be a "promising element" (Norcross, 2002) for study in the effectiveness of psychotherapy. It is considered to be integral to the helping relationship which is known to be a highly effective component of therapeutic practice (Audet & Everall, 2003; Hill & Knox, 2001; Knox & Hill, 2003). The professional literature also generally reflects a positive view of self-disclosure (Audet & Everall, 2003). Where differences exist is the purpose and nature of the disclosure.

The purpose of self-disclosure is an important consideration. Use to further the therapy process or assistance to a particular client is justifiable. When it is for the therapist's benefit, such as a desire for closeness or compliments, it is not easily defended (Pietkiewicz & Skowrońska-Włoch, 2017). This distinction lies with the therapist's judgment as well as the client's judgment. The client's judgment is essential and requires sensitivity by the therapist to determine and respect. It need not be limited to specific types, behaviors, and actions, but rather the totality of what a client learns about the relationship and their therapist (Pietkiewicz & Skowrońska-Włoch, 2017).

Different types of self-disclosure exist. These fall into categories such as facts and feelings, insight and strategy, and support and challenge (Pietkiewicz & Skowrońska-Włoch, 2017). Another distinction is between intentional and unintentional. Unintentional self-disclosure may be apparent in reactions to difficult topics such as sexuality, religion, or politics, as well as unavoidable evidenced by age or possibly ethnicity and abilities. Self-disclosure may be evident in the therapy setting itself (artwork, music, for example) and directly telling a client something (Pietkiewicz & Skowrońska-Włoch, 2017). Another possibly unintentional self-disclosure may occur through a virtual or online presence by the therapist as a professional or private citizen.

Professional and personal disclosure are different from each other. Professional information may include education and experience as well as regulatory and professional memberships. Personal information concerns most everything else. The former requires little reflection on the part of the therapist while the latter certainly does. Interpersonal disclosure, which is also called immediacy, concerns the relationship between the client and therapist in the present moment (Audet, 2011). While potentially beneficial, the sharing of information can alter the boundaries between therapist and client. Such a change can potentially confuse a client about their role and in extreme circumstances, lead to caregiving toward the therapist (Audet & Everall, 2003). Indeed Barnett (1998) cautions that "the sharing of personal material by the counselor could alter the client's expectations of psychotherapy and the process of psychotherapy and therefore must be done with great care" (p. 421) (Audet & Everall, 2003). If this occurs in an online context, the therapist may not know what the client does or does not already know about them (Bratt, 2010).

Consider your boundaries about your use of social media. Do you maintain separate professional and personal pages and usernames? Do you have an integrated online presence? What are the pros and cons of each? How do you protect your privacy while advertising your services?

Dual Relationships

A dual relationship is the addition of a nontherapeutic relationship to an existing therapeutic relationship with a client. It is becoming recognized that in some settings, such as rural or remote, or communities, such as Indigenous or LGBTQ2+ communities, those other relationships with clients are not always avoidable. The nature of these relationships varies from intimate relations and others that benefit the therapist also in either tangible ways (e.g. investment advice) and nonmaterial or emotional ways (e.g. a friendship) (Reamer, 1998). They may also be motivated by a therapist's altruism to assist clients in ways outside of their usual roles (e.g. advocate on a client's behalf with their landlord). Finally, there are unexpected encounters with clients in other settings (Pugh, 2006). The potential for harm to a client is an essential criterion for considering risk about the potential benefit (Hartmann, 1997). The onus is on the therapist to ensure that the conflict of interest created by such an arrangement does not do any harm (Pietkiewicz & Skowrońska-Włoch, 2017).

Some dual relationships are not avoidable. For example, a therapist and client may find out that they have some common friends or associates (Lazarus & Zur, 2002). In small communities, especially, the therapist is more visible and identifiable (Pugh, 2006). A more informal style of relating is potentially a part of the local culture and as such, the higher likelihood that a client wants to situate the therapist with others that the client knows (Pugh, 2006).

Another type of dual relationship is an online relationship as well as in person. These may or may not involve different roles. In either case, there is potential for the professional therapeutic relationship to become widened or distorted. Online relationships with clients may not always be evident to a therapist who has been friended on Facebook or followed on snap chat. Clients may seek out their therapists online to learn more about them or become connected as an extension of the professional relationship or within the therapists knowing (Bratt, 2010).

Think about the potential for dual relationships in your community. What would you do if your client is also your server at a restaurant? What if your client is a store clerk and packing your groceries? Mechanic for your car? Your pharmacist?

Decision-Making

There are several factors to consider in decisions concerning boundaries. The extent to which cultural diversity is relevant may be indicated by the judgment the client makes about the appropriateness of a comment or action. For example, a young therapist referring to a client in their 50s as "old". Is shaking the hand of a client appropriate only if the client extends their hand first (in order to determine if handshaking is acceptable to a client)? (Barnett, 2015). The therapists' discomfort with a behavior despite a client's explicit request is also an important criterion (e.g. being asked for a hug from a client). The theoretical orientation of the therapist and nature of therapy may also play a role (e.g. systematic desensitization training by meeting a client in public setting) (Gabbard, 2001).

Cognitive errors that therapists may make concerning decisions about boundaries with clients have been identified (Pope and Keith-Spiegel, 2008). Error 1: What Happens Outside the Psychotherapy Session Has Nothing to Do with the therapy (e.g. joining a public group to which the client belongs and determining that because it takes place outside of the clinical encounter that it is not related to the therapy). Error 2: Crossing a Boundary with a Therapy Client Has the Same Meaning as Doing the Same Thing With Someone Who Is Not a Client (e.g. out of basic courtesy, giving a client a ride). Error 3: Our Understanding of a Boundary Crossing Is Also the Client's Understanding of the Boundary Crossing (e.g. telling a client that they look very "put together"). Error 4: A Boundary Crossing That Is Therapeutic for One Client Also Will Be Therapeutic for Another Client This (e.g. the preceding example, and a different client's positive reaction). Error 5: A Boundary Crossing Is a Static, Isolated Event (e.g. the lingering effect of a comment that took a client by surprise or offense). Error 6: If We Do Not See Any Self-Interest, Problems, Conflicts of Interest, Unintended Consequences, Major Risks, or Potential Downsides to Crossing a Particular Boundary, Then There Are Not Any. We may not see things objectively enough at the moment. Error 7 Self-Disclosure Is, Per Se, Always Therapeutic Because It Shows Authenticity, Transparency, and Trust. Not necessarily. It may not have value for the therapy (Pope & Keith-Spiegel, 2008).

Addressing Missteps

Once a boundary crossing occurs, and there is evidence that it was less helpful than harmful to the client, the therapist may work through it, if appropriate, with the client. However, if the matter is highly sensitive, such as in the case of sexual attraction, this would be done in supervision and not with a client.

A process described by therapists about their own experience of attraction to a client started with recognizing and taking personal responsibility, reflecting and making sense of the experience, and proceeding with what is in the client's best interest (Martin, Godfrey, Meekums, & Madill, 2011). Awareness that something was amiss occurred through self- monitoring and recognition of more extreme reaction than usual. Potential reactions of shame or guilt may be barriers or motivators to address the issue.

Reflecting on the issue and reactions to it may also be instructive about what the therapist is bringing to the situation and which personal vulnerabilities are in play—making sense of the situation, themselves and their role within the context of immediate personal pressures affecting them and in need of management. "The final steps involved sense-making in terms of the client's issues and working out ways of returning to therapeutic work, using the situation, if possible, for the client's benefit" (Martin et al., 2011).

SUMMARY

- The wounded healer refers to the connection that woundedness for the therapist and client each separately have experienced. The therapist, having progressed along with their healing, is positioned to assist a client to explore and heal. It is a process of compassion that flows from therapist to client and then back to the therapist.
- Woundedness can provide a commonality of experience. Such openness by a therapist may decrease the distance and power differential.
- Boundaries concern the regulations that therapists are to comply with about who will do what when. They describe what is out of bounds and separate the professional relationship from others.
- A crossing can be justified clinically, concerning a particular theory or activity, specific need or exceptional circumstance, while a violation is done more about an exceptional need of the therapist.

DISCUSSION QUESTIONS

1. How is it possible for a therapists woundedness, if not well-managed, to become a boundary problem? What wounds? What boundaries? What is your theory of the relationship between the two?

2. How will you manage your personal and professional presence on social media? Will you keep them separate or integrated? What are the pros and cons of each?
3. Which are the most likely boundary challenges you will experience? How will you recognize your boundary challenges? How can you take preventive action? How can you take remedial action?

REFERENCES

Audet, C. T. (2011). Client perspectives of therapist self-disclosure: Violating boundaries or removing barriers? *Counselling Psychology Quarterly, 24*(2), 85–100.

Audet, C., & Everall, R. D. (2003). Counsellor self-disclosure: Client-informed implications for practice. *Counselling and Psychotherapy Research, 3*(3), 223–231.

Austin, W., Bergum, V., Nuttgens, S., & Peternelj-Taylor, C. (2006). A re-visioning of boundaries in professional helping relationships: Exploring other metaphors. *Ethics and Behavior, 16*(2), 77–94.

Barnett, J. E. (1998). Should psychotherapists self-disclose? Clinical and ethical considerations. In L. Vandecreek, S. Knapp, & T. L. Jackson (Eds.), *Innovations in clinical practice: A source book.* Sarasota, FL: Professional Resource Exchange.

Barnett, J. E. (2015). A practical ethics approach to boundaries and multiple relationships in psychotherapy. *British Psychological Society Psychotherapy Section Review, 56*(1), 27–37.

Bojuwoye, O. (2001). Crossing cultural boundaries in counselling. *International Journal for the Advancement of Counselling, 23*(1), 31–50.

Bratt, W. E. V. (2010). Ethical considerations of social networking for counsellors. *Canadian Journal of Counselling and Psychotherapy, 44*(4), 335–345.

Bridges, N. A. (1999). Psychodynamic perspective on therapeutic boundaries: Creative clinical possibilities. *The Journal of Psychotherapy Practice and Research, 8*(4), 292.

Conti-O'Hare, M. (1998). Examining the wounded healer archetype: A case study in expert addictions nursing practice. *Journal of the American Psychiatric Nurses Association, 4*(3), 71–76.

Dindia, K., & Allen, M. (1992). Sex differences in self-disclosure: A meta-analysis. *Psychological Bulletin, 112*(1), 106–124.

Dorpat, T. L. (1977). On neutrality. *International Journal of Psychoanalytic Psychotherapy, 6,* 39–64.

Gabbard, G. O. (1996). Lessons to be learned from the study of sexual boundary violations. *American Journal of Psychotherapy, 50*(3), 311–322.

Gabbard, G. O. (2001). Commentary: Boundaries, culture, and psychotherapy. *Journal of the American Academy of Psychiatry and the Law Online, 29*(3), 284–286.

Groesbeck, C. J. (1975). The archetypal image of the wounded healer. *Journal of Analytical Psychology, 20*(2), 122–145.

Gutheil, T. G., & Gabbard, G. O. (1998). Misuses and misunderstandings of boundary theory in clinical and regulatory settings. *American Journal of Psychiatry, 155*(3), 409–414.

Hanshew, E. R. (1998, April). An investigation of the wounded healer phenomenon: Counselor trainees and their self-conscious emotions and mental health. *Dissertation Abstracts International, 58*(10-A), 3846, US: University Microfilms International.

Hartmann, E. (1997). The concept of boundaries in counselling and psychotherapy. *British Journal of Guidance and Counselling, 25*(2), 147–162.

Hay, J. (2018). Psychological boundaries and psychological bridges: A categorisation and the application of transactional analysis concepts. *International Journal of Transactional Analysis Research & Practice, 9*(1), 52–81.

Hermansson, G. (1997). Boundaries and boundary management in counselling: The never-ending story. *British Journal of Guidance and Counselling, 25*(2), 133–146.

Heru, A. M., Strong, D., Price, M., & Recupero, P. R. (2006). Self-disclosure in psychotherapy supervisors: Gender differences. *American Journal of Psychotherapy, 60*(4), 323–334.

Hill, C. E., & Knox, S. (2001). Self-disclosure. *Psychotherapy: Theory, Research, Practice, Training, 38*(4), 413.

Jung, C. G. (1951). Fundamental questions of psychotherapy. *Collected Works, 16,* 116.

Jung, C. G., & Jung, C. G. J. (1963). *Memories, dreams, reflections* (Vol. 268). New York: Vintage.

Kirmayer, L. J. (2003). Asklepian dreams: The ethos of the wounded-healer in the clinical encounter. *Transcultural Psychiatry, 40*(2), 248–277.

Knapp, S., & Slattery, J. M. (2004). Professional boundaries in nontraditional settings. *Professional Psychology: Research and Practice, 35*(5), 553.

Knox, S., & Hill, C. E. (2003). Therapist self-disclosure: Research-based suggestions for practitioners. *Journal of Clinical Psychology, 59*(5), 529–539.

Laskowski, C., & Pellicore, K. (2002). The wounded healer archetype: Applications to palliative care practice. *American Journal of Hospice and Palliative Medicine®, 19*(6), 403–407.

Laungani, P. (2004). Counselling and therapy in a multi-cultural setting. *Counselling Psychology Quarterly, 17*(2), 195–207.

Lazarus, A. A., & Zur, O. (2002). *Dual relationships and psychotherapy.* New York, NY: Springer.

Martin, C., Godfrey, M., Meekums, B., & Madill, A. (2011). Managing boundaries under pressure: A qualitative study of therapists' experiences of sexual attraction in therapy. *Counselling and Psychotherapy Research, 11*(4), 248–256.

Montgomery, J. D. (1991). *Social networks and persistent inequality in the labor market*. Evanston: Center for Urban Affairs and Policy Research.

Norcross, J. C. (2002). *Psychotherapy relationships that work: Therapist contributions and responsiveness to patients*. New York: Oxford University Press.

Owen, I. R. (1997). Boundaries in the practice of humanistic counselling. *British Journal of Guidance and Counselling, 25*(2), 163–174.

Pietkiewicz, I., & Skowrońska-Włoch, K. (2017). Attitudes to professional boundaries among therapists with and without substance abuse history. *Polish Psychological Bulletin, 48*(3), 411–422.

Pope, K. S., & Keith-Spiegel, P. (2008). A practical approach to boundaries in psychotherapy: Making decisions, bypassing blunders, and mending fences. *Journal of Clinical Psychology, 64*(5), 638–652.

Pugh, R. (2006). Dual relationships: Personal and professional boundaries in rural social work. *British Journal of Social Work, 37*(8), 1405–1423.

Reamer, F. G. (1998). The evolution of social work ethics. *Social Work, 43*(6), 488–500.

Searles, H. (1975). The patient as therapist to his analyst. In P. Giovacchini (Ed.), *Classics in psychoanalytic technique* (pp. 103–138). New York: Jason Arsonson.

Sedgwick, D. (1994). *The wounded healer: Countertransference from a Jungian perspective*. London: Routledge.

Sedgwick, D. (2016). *The wounded healer: Countertransference from a Jungian perspective*. London: Routledge.

Smith, D., & Fitzpatrick, M. (1995). Patient-therapist boundary issues: An integrative review of theory and research. *Professional Psychology: Research and Practice, 26*(5), 499.

Stone, D. (2008). Wounded healing: Exploring the circle of compassion in the helping relationship. *The Humanistic Psychologist, 36*(1), 45–51.

Westergaard, J. (2013). Counselling young people: Counsellors' perspectives on 'what works'—An exploratory study. *Counselling and Psychotherapy Research, 13*(2), 98–105.

Zerubavel, N., & Wright, M. O. D. (2012). The dilemma of the wounded healer. *Psychotherapy, 49*(4), 482.

CHAPTER 9

Caring and Coping

The very qualities that contribute to therapist effectiveness have the potential to lead to fatigue and burnout (Thompson, Amatea, & Thompson, 2014). Fortunately, there have been many documented means by which therapists can frame and manage challenges. This chapter includes a discussion of the nature and impact of compassion in therapy and its effects on therapists (Marriage & Marriage, 2005). Stress associated with more global experiences of the therapy work in the context of the workplace and its demands occurs before reviews of study results identifying ways therapists restore a sense of self and balance.

Compassion

Compassion in counseling and psychotherapy is often associated with mindfulness and its connections to Buddhist philosophy. Research on mindfulness is becoming well developed, while research on compassion is limited (Elices et al., 2017). However, there has been a great deal of attention paid to compassion-related injuries associated with traumatic experiences clients discuss in therapy and their effects on therapists who have or have not had traumatic experiences of their own. Stress and coping are concepts that have garnered a fair degree of interest with factors leading to burnout having a prominent place in the professional literature.

© The Author(s) 2019   143
J. D. Brown, *Reflective Practice of Counseling and Psychotherapy in a Diverse Society*, https://doi.org/10.1007/978-3-030-24505-4_9

Compassion translates from Latin, where it means "to suffer with" (Strauss et al., 2016). Buddhist psychology takes it to mean that one is both in touch with suffering in self and others as well as committed to relief from suffering (Lama & Thupten, 1995; Neff, 2003). The four processes include cognitive, affective, intention, and motivation (Jazaieri et al., 2013). It is not necessarily directed toward self or specific others, but to all of humanity (Elices et al., 2017).

From both evolutionary and biological perspectives, compassion has an adaptive purpose. The care for one's children is a biologically predisposed and evolutionary necessity. This care for one's own extends to care for others beyond extended family and alliance members (Barrett, Dunbar, & Lycett, 2002), which may include strangers and nonhumans (Gilbert, 2015). Payoffs include adaptation and survival expression (Slavich & Cole, 2013). Recent studies have found psychological benefits as well as beneficial social relationships to be associated with compassion (Gilbert, 2015; Jazaieri et al., 2013).

An inclusive definition of compassion represents five qualities (Strauss et al., 2016). These qualities include (1) recognition of suffering, (2) appreciating the universality of suffering, (3) empathy with those who are suffering and feeling connected to it, as well as (4) tolerating the discomfort in order to accept the person, and (5) taking action to alleviate it (Elices et al., 2017).

Taking the perspective of another and tolerating the unpleasantness or discomfort of the suffering are essential capacities (Gilbert, 2015). A model of dimensions, or types of compassion (Ekman, 2014), includes empathetic compassion, action compassion, concerned compassion, and aspirational compassion. Concern for others' welfare with an aspiration of alleviating collective suffering provides a context within which everyone is worthy (Gilbert, 2015). Despite disliking another person, it is possible to feel compassion for them.

While the courage to enter into the suffering of others is noble, but without the knowledge to assist, the outcome is that both suffer together (Germer & Siegel, 2012). Another important distinction is between doing for someone and doing with someone. The compassion that results in doing for can be helpful but leaves the recipient in a position of requiring another to assist if the problem reoccurs. In contrast, doing with shows how to reduce suffering so that the client knows how to help themselves (Gilbert, 2015).

Is compassion necessary in therapy? Does it assist the therapist? Does it assist the client? Is there a point at which it is too much for a client? As a therapist, how would you know when your client is pushing away the compassion you attempt to share? Why might that be? How would you know when you are feeling too little or too much compassion?

Self-Compassion

There is emerging evidence that compassion toward others and self are distinct (Neff & Pommier, 2013). Self-compassion means to care for self as one would care for another, which includes suspending judgment and feeling one's suffering (Elices et al., 2017). Self-compassion is not a selfish act, but rather an extension of the awareness that all are deserving of compassion, including oneself and no one is above the need for compassion (Neff & Seppälä, 2016). Neff (2003) refers to this aspect as our shared humanity. Three significant components of self-compassion are self-judgment versus self-kindness, feelings of isolation versus a sense of common humanity, and over-identification versus mindfulness (Neff, 2003).

Barriers to Compassion

Compassion can stall due to a variety of internal and external, emotional and social obstructions and barriers (Gilbert, 2015). Why might one choose to avoid compassion? Maintain separation of self? Concern about vulnerability and contagion?

What appears to be compassion from an observation might be motivated by a need or want that is not to alleviate another's suffering for that person's benefit. For example, one may show consideration and caring to avoid being put on the spot because of a fear of being rejected.

Compassionate behavior toward others in order to fit in does not carry the benefits of self-compassion that includes both self-acceptance and self-care. It is associated with higher levels of stress, worries, and sadness (Gilbert, 2005). In another example, the competing needs for caring and survival, helping versus hindering, can play out where the self takes precedence over all others. Compassion, in such a setting, can be turned off (Zimbardo & Boyd, 2008).

Avoidance of compassion may be an adaptive response to the overwhelming cruelty and violence, injustice and distress evident in the media and personal experience. Staying within one's own small family or community and disassociating from those who are outside can be self-protective. It also allows for immense suffering to continue, unaffected (Gilbert & Mascaro, 2017). It can be justified by placing blame on the others or relegating others to groups that are less worthy (Skitka, 1999). However, failure to resist immoral authority can result in incredible cruelty (Kelman & Hamilton, 1989).

> Are there times when your self-compassion needs nurturing? How do you know? Can you show compassion to others if you do not have it for yourself? How is this possible?

Compassion Fatigue

Compassion is a fundamental part of counseling and psychotherapy. The benefits of feeling cared for, engaged with, and helped by having effects on the relationship and therapy progress (Crocker & Canevello, 2012; Gilbert, 2005). Compassion as a central focus for intervention is showing evidence of effectiveness (Hofmann, Grossman, & Hinton, 2011). Compassion for self and others is associated with more optimal functioning (Cacioppo & Patrick, 2008), but for therapists, it comes with emotional costs. Depletion, regression, and injury are possible results of working with clients who have experienced trauma. These effects manifest as vicarious traumatization, secondary traumatic stress, and compassion fatigue (Sodeke-Gregson, Holttum, & Billings, 2013).

Secondary traumatic stress is acute. It has a rapid onset and includes symptoms similar to post-traumatic stress disorder (Newell & MacNeil, 2010). It has been defined as the "natural and consequential behaviors and emotions resulting from knowing about a traumatizing event experienced by a significant other [or client] and the stress resulting from helping or wanting to help a traumatized or suffering person [or client]" (Figley, 1995, p. 7). Descriptions focus more on the outward signs than the internal cognitive and emotional processes involved (Newell & MacNeil, 2010).

Vicarious traumatization develops over time and exposure to traumatic experiences presented by clients (Newell & MacNeil, 2010). The effects are associated with the alteration of one's frame of reference and thus, cognitive and emotional (Sodeke-Gregson et al., 2013). It is a fundamental alteration in "sense of self, world view, spirituality, affect tolerance, interpersonal relationships, and imagery system of memory" (Pearlman, 1999, p. 52). The basis of beliefs of a world in which the therapist has safety, trust, and control for those who have vicarious traumatization are challenged and brought into question (Newell & MacNeil, 2010).

Traumatic Countertransference

Countertransference may be distinguished from compassion fatigue as the cumulative effects of exposure on the therapist over time versus a single instance, as is the case for countertransference (Sodeke-Gregson et al., 2013). They overlap insofar as the traumatic experience of a client transfers to the therapist and that across cases shared qualities (e.g. victim-victimizer-bystander) emerge (Berzoff & Kita, 2010).

The cumulative effects of compassion fatigue may manifest behaviorally, emotionally and cognitively (Figley, 2002). Impatience and irritation, hypervigilance, memory loss, and nightmares may be present. Feelings of guilt, powerlessness and rage and fear, as well as depletion, may occur. Cognitive effects may include apathy, negativity, depersonalization, and preoccupation with the trauma (Berzoff & Kita, 2010). Compassion fatigue can alter the therapists' sense of meaning and hope and in doing so, affect the potential for useful and helpful countertransference (Berzoff & Kita, 2010).

When a therapist's own traumatic experience is triggered or awakened through the process of therapy with a client who has experienced trauma, the product may be traumatic countertransference (Herman & Harvey, 1997). In such cases, the support of another clinician or team to assist the therapist to identify the clients' reality and distinguish it from their own experience can be invaluable (Berzoff & Kita, 2010). Compassion fatigue may be reduced through the adoption of a more balanced life-style, while countertransference requires personal exploration and engagement with one's trauma (Hafkenscheid, 2005).

STRESS AND BURNOUT

Stress is the product of the perceived demands of a situation requiring exceeding the resources one possesses. The experience of the same situation varies considerably across cognitive, emotional, physiological, and interpersonal processes that include: an appraisal of the situation, perceived coping strategies, and the commensurate resources needed (Pakenham & Stafford-Brown, 2012). Lazarus and Folkman's definition from 1984 remains influential today, where stress is "a relationship between the person and the environment that is appraised by the person as taxing or exceeding his or her resources and endangering his or her well-being" (p. 19).

Burnout includes the perceptions of stress held by the individual (Gam, Kim, & Jeon, 2016). It is a phenomenon not associated necessarily with a traumatic experience, but rather the global demands of a situation. It encompasses the entire work experience and context with development over the longer term and perception of little to no likelihood for change (Awa, Plaumann, & Walter, 2010). The three qualities of burnout include emotional exhaustion (emotional and physical depletion), depersonalization (increased emotional distance from clients), and personal accomplishment (low levels of satisfaction and ability) (Maslach & Goldberg, 1998).

The qualities of emotional exhaustion and depersonalization have been the subject of research on therapists' experiences of stress and coping. Emotional exhaustion is associated with low control and high overinvolvement, low job satisfaction as well as younger age, long hours of work, and the work setting (Lee, Lim, Yang, & Lee, 2011). Depersonalization is associated with younger age, male gender, fewer years of work experience, long work hours, and settings (Lim, Kim, Kim, Yang, & Lee, 2010).

Burnout occurs over time and is the result of the cumulative effects of stress. The effects have a gradual effect on the quality of service provided and become increasingly noticeable (Lee et al., 2011). Contributing factors are apparent in populations served, and the organizations within which one works (Maslach, 2001, 2003a, b). Organizational structures and job pressures, overload, role conflict, and ambiguity are contributors (Marriage & Marriage, 2005). The most significant single risk factor is human service work (Newell & MacNeil, 2010). Effects include relationship breakdowns, early retirement, reduced performance, mental and physical health challenges, as well as substance misuse (Marriage & Marriage, 2005).

What signals that tell you that your level of stress is high? What do you do in those circumstances? Are there times you had practiced when you were not at your best? How suboptimal can you be and continue to practice safely? How do you know when you need to take action to manage stress? What might you notice in a coworker struggling with stress? At what point would you consider it to have become problematic? What would you do? Why?

Growth-Oriented Coping

Increasing attention is focusing on positive aspects of trauma-related and work-related stress. While challenges are inevitable, there is potential for personal growth as a result of stress. Three concepts that appear in the literature include compassion satisfaction, vicarious resilience, and thriving.

Have you ever felt encouraged by the work you do? How is it possible to feel good about being with others in times of pain and suffering? What does it mean to you to have a sense of fulfillment from your work? How do you maintain this?

Compassion satisfaction has been defined by Larsen and Stamm (2008) as "the sense of fulfilment or pleasure that therapists derive from doing their work well" (p. 282). It includes the satisfaction received from the work, how competent one feels, being insufficient control of one's processing through therapy, and levels of support including both structural and functional (Sodeke-Gregson et al., 2013).

Vicarious resilience emerged from research on the personal changes occurring as a result of a therapist's exposure to traumatic experiences of their clients. Therapists identified the necessity of finding purpose in work and meaning in their lives. For some therapists, the challenges encountered that resulted in their change created strategies and ways of operating that helped them find strength and resilience. "This immersion in trauma, paradoxically, enhanced the participants' ability to 'bounce back' or buffer the more negative effects of the work" (Pack, 2014). The importance of managing the dissonance created from hearing about traumatic experiences while living a life where freedom from the fear that accompanies one's vulnerability is a necessity for their relationships to be healthy.

Qualities that facilitated this process include empathetic engagement (to appreciate another's experience), a "search for self" and a "search beyond self." This process creates meaning for the therapist of self concerning others and clients via spiritual meaning and purpose (Pack, 2014). It also permits the coexistence of relationships with others, including professionals and the social context within which therapy for traumatic experience is needed and necessary (Pack, 2014).

Thriving as a concept refers to the move past simply coping, to fuller engagement and meaning within the context of one's work. All experience, from such a view, is an opportunity to learn and contribute (Spreitzer, Sutcliffe, Dutton, Sonenshein, & Grant, 2005). Three forces that are associated with this experience include control, relationships, and meaning (Sim, Zanardelli, Loughran, Mannarino, & Hill, 2016). Autonomy and decision-making power are reflected in control while being appreciated and appreciating others at work are central to relationships (Spreitzer et al., 2005). Feeling a sense of purpose for the work and one's place in it is central to a sense of meaning (Nielsen & Einarsen, 2012). These forces can be enhanced through an examination of the work environment, interpersonal relationships, tasks within the workplace, involvement with professional associations, and personal coping strategies (Sim et al., 2016).

Meaning-Oriented Coping

As highlighted within the growth-oriented approaches, a sense of purpose and meaning for therapists may be central to the maintenance of healthy functioning in their role and workplace (as well as family and community).

The humanist and existential traditions centralize the importance of meaning, but the meaning may also be a function of cognitive restructuring. Attribution allows for the creation or adoption of an explanation when there is no adequate explanation (Malle, 2011). It is one means by which meaning can be attached to the experience and through the accumulation of experiences, a more cohesive view may emerge.

Humor, based on a critical or witty reframing of a painful experience to create some distance from the topic and release of tension, is also successfully employed as a way of coping (Moran, 2002). Also, there is evidence that sense of self as a spiritual person is also a way of appreciating the bigger picture within which one is a part (Hardiman & Simmonds, 2013). Coping may utilize increased "attention to metaphysical and existential questions, such as the meaning and purpose of life, the nature of one's existence, the existence of a God or higher power, one's personal spirituality" (Hardiman & Simmonds, 2013). Some studies that have investigated trauma coping and health have presented evidence in support of the importance of spirituality for therapists (Jones, Topping, Wattis, & Smith, 2016).

Attribution is a style of interpretation and pattern creation that can help reframe stressful experiences (Peterson et al., 1982). As a style, attribution includes attention to three dimensions (Lee et al., 2018). Internal versus external refers to the extent to which an event occurs because of an inside or outside force. Stable versus unstable refers to the cause of the event changes or remains consistent. Finally, global versus specific refers to the cause as a generalizable one or one that is highly specific to that particular event. In response to an adverse event, a pessimistic view might identify the causes as internal, stable, and global, while an optimistic view might identify the causes as external, unstable, and specific (Lee et al., 2018).

> Consider a recent event in your personal or professional life that was stressful. Explore what happened from different attributional styles of internal versus external, stable versus unstable, global versus specific. Note any differences in how you view and feel about it comparing the way (1) you experienced it and the way (2) you reframed it with the opposite attributions.

Self-Protective Coping

Most coping research that applies to professionals in counseling and psychotherapy refers to specific strategies used by therapists to manage their exposure to trauma and stress from their clients and their workplace. One theory that continues to garner attention is the distinction between problem-focused and emotion-focused coping (Folkman & Lazarus, 1980). Problem-focused coping is active. Its purpose is to address the situation directly. It is useful, however, when there is no, and it is within the persons means to do it. Emotion-focused coping is passive. Its purpose is to avoid or accept the situation. It is useful when there is nothing that can be done or at least nothing that the individual can do about the situation. While some data suggest that therapists choose activities of both types, therapists in private practice tend to use more problem-focused coping than therapists in organizations use more emotion-focused coping (Sim et al., 2016).

The strategies reported by therapists exist in three categories. Personal strategies are not dependent on the profession or workplace and apply primarily to what one has control over in their personal life. Professional strategies are within the role of a therapist as a professional providing a recognized and regulated service. Finally, organizational strategies are those that are within the workplace itself.

Personal strategies may include (e.g. Sim et al., 2016).

- Physical activities and exercise
- Interpersonal support (friends, activities)
- Creating distinctions between home/personal time and work/professional time
- Engaging in acts of kindness
- Spiritual practices
- Limiting exposure to trauma (avoiding media violence)
- Relaxation and meditation
- Nutrition, sleep, recreation
- Drawing, painting, cooking
- Psychotherapy
- Detachment
- Positive outlook

Professional strategies may include (e.g. Lakey & Cohen, 2000; Newell & MacNeil, 2010):

- Experience to recognize issues and relationships
- Learning about different professional topics
- Rituals at the beginning and end of sessions
- Planning and taking holidays and vacations
- Becoming an advocate
- Cultivating coworker support and teamwork
- Delegating
- Professional peer supervision

Organizational strategies may include (Newell & MacNeil, 2010):

- Formal and informal debriefing
- Peer support
- Workload management
- Goal setting
- Breaks
- Employee assistance
- Demand reduction
- Autonomy-enhancing
- Balanced decision-making

Students of psychotherapy and counseling describe the main barriers to the utilization of a range of coping strategies (El-Ghoroury, Galper, Sawaqder, & Bufka, 2012). The barriers reported were lack of time, cannot afford/ financial constraints, worry about what could happen, lack of motivation, energy, or interest, shame, guilt, or embarrassment, privacy and or confidentiality concerns, don't know about available resources, inadequate social support, discouragement or hopelessness, minimization or denial of problem, fear of loss of professional status, and fear of licensing board actions.

Do any of the coping strategies or barriers listed here apply to you? Which ones? Are there any other forms of coping that you have found helpful? What are they? What makes them helpful? Which barriers are the strongest for you? What are some ways to overcome them?

SUMMARY

- Internal and external factors, emotional and social obstructions and barriers affect the experience of compassion.
- Secondary traumatic stress is acute. It has a rapid onset and includes symptoms similar to post-traumatic stress disorder. Vicarious traumatization develops over time and exposure to traumatic experiences presented by clients.
- Stress is the perceived demands of a situation above accessible resources. While the objective characteristics of the situation may be consistent, the experience of that situation may vary considerably across individuals. Burnout concerns the perceptions of stress held by the individual. It encompasses the entire work experience and context with development over the longer term and perception of little to no likelihood for change.
- Increasing attention focuses on positive aspects of trauma-related and work-related stress. Three concepts that appear in the literature include compassion satisfaction, vicarious resilience, and thriving.

DISCUSSION QUESTIONS

1. Is it inappropriate for therapists to care for themselves through their care for clients? Why? How do therapists benefit emotionally from their practice?
2. How much more should a therapist care about a client than the client cares about themselves? What are the limits on this? How do you know when you have reached a limit? How do you cope with having done all you can, and a client has not found improvement?
3. How can therapists protect themselves from the traumatic experiences of their clients? Are there times when letting your guard down necessary to be helpful to a client? In what ways? How far down?

REFERENCES

Awa, W. L., Plaumann, M., & Walter, U. (2010). Burnout prevention: A review of intervention programs. *Patient Education and Counseling, 78*(2), 184–190.

Barrett, L., Dunbar, R., & Lycett, J. (2002). *Human evolutionary psychology.* Princeton: Princeton University Press.

Berzoff, J., & Kita, E. (2010). Compassion fatigue and countertransference: Two different concepts. *Clinical Social Work Journal, 38*(3), 341–349.

Cacioppo, J. T., & Patrick, W. (2008). *Loneliness: Human nature and the need for social connection*. New York: W. W. Norton.

Crocker, J., & Canevello, A. (2012). Consequences of self-image and compassionate goals. In *Advances in experimental social psychology* (Vol. 45, pp. 229–277). Amsterdam: Academic Press.

Ekman, P. (2014). *Moving toward global compassion*. New York: Author.

El-Ghoroury, N. H., Galper, D. I., Sawaqdeh, A., & Bufka, L. F. (2012). Stress, coping, and barriers to wellness among psychology graduate students. *Training and Education in Professional Psychology, 6*(2), 122.

Elices, M., Carmona, C., Pascual, J. C., Feliu-Soler, A., Martin-Blanco, A., & Soler, J. (2017). Compassion and self-compassion: Construct and measurement. *Mindfulness & Compassion, 2*(1), 34–40.

Figley, C. R. (1995). *Compassion fatigue: Coping with secondary traumatic stress disorder in those who treat the traumatized*. Levittown, PA: Brunner/Mazel.

Figley, C. R. (2002). Compassion fatigue: Psychotherapists' chronic lack of self care. *Journal of Clinical Psychology, 58*(11), 1433–1441.

Folkman, S., & Lazarus, R. S. (1980). An analysis of coping in a middle-aged community sample. *Journal of Health and Social Behavior, 21*, 219–239.

Gam, J., Kim, G., & Jeon, Y. (2016). Influences of art therapists' self-efficacy and stress coping strategies on burnout. *The Arts in Psychotherapy, 47*, 1–8.

Germer, C. K., & Siegel, R. D. (Eds.). (2012). *Wisdom and compassion in psychotherapy: Deepening mindfulness in clinical practice*. New York: Guilford Press.

Gilbert, P. (Ed.). (2005). *Compassion: Conceptualisations, research and use in psychotherapy*. New York: Routledge.

Gilbert, P. (2015). The evolution and social dynamics of compassion. *Social and Personality Psychology Compass, 9*(6), 239–254.

Gilbert, P., & Mascaro, J. (2017). Compassion: Fears, blocks, and resistances: An evolutionary investigation. In *The Oxford handbook of compassion science* (pp. 391–418). Oxford: Oxford University Press.

Hafkenscheid, A. (2005). Event countertransference and vicarious traumatization: Theoretically valid and clinically useful concepts? *European Journal of Psychotherapy & Counselling, 7*(3), 159–168.

Hardiman, P., & Simmonds, J. G. (2013). Spiritual well-being, burnout and trauma in counsellors and psychotherapists. *Mental Health, Religion & Culture, 16*(10), 1044–1055.

Herman, J. L., & Harvey, M. R. (1997). Adult memories of childhood trauma: A naturalistic clinical study. *Journal of Traumatic Stress, 10*(4), 557–571.

Hofmann, S. G., Grossman, P., & Hinton, D. E. (2011). Loving-kindness and compassion meditation: Potential for psychological interventions. *Clinical Psychology Review, 31*, 1126–1132.

Jazaieri, H., Jinpa, G. T., McGonigal, K., Rosenberg, E. L., Finkelstein, J., Simon-Thomas, E., ... Goldin, P. R. (2013). Enhancing compassion: A randomized controlled trial of a compassion cultivation training program. *Journal of Happiness Studies*, *14*(4), 1113–1126.

Jones, J., Topping, A., Wattis, J., & Smith, J. (2016). A concept analysis of spirituality in occupational therapy practice. *Journal for the Study of Spirituality*, *6*(1), 38–57.

Kelman, H. C., & Hamilton, V. L. (1989). *Crimes of obedience: Toward a social psychology of authority and responsibility*. New Haven: Yale University Press.

Lakey, B., & Cohen, S. (2000). Social support and theory. In *Social support measurement and intervention: A guide for health and social scientists* (p. 29). Oxford: Oxford University Press.

Lama, D., & Thupten, J. (1995). *The power of compassion*. New Delhi, India: HarperCollins.

Larsen, D., & Stamm, B. H. (2008). Professional quality of life and trauma therapists. In S. Joseph & P. A. Linley (Eds.), *Trauma, recovery, and growth: Positive psychological perspectives on posttraumatic stress* (pp. 275–293). Hoboken, NJ: Wiley.

Lee, I., Bardhoshi, G., Yoon, E., Sandersfeld, T., Rush, R. D., & Priest, J. B. (2018). Attributional style and burnout of counselors-in-training. *Counselor Education and Supervision*, *57*(4), 285–300.

Lee, J., Lim, N., Yang, E., & Lee, S. M. (2011). Antecedents and consequences of three dimensions of burnout in psychotherapists: A meta-analysis. *Professional Psychology: Research and Practice*, *42*(3), 252.

Lim, N., Kim, E. K., Kim, H., Yang, E., & Lee, S. M. (2010). Individual and work-related factors influencing burnout of mental health professionals: A meta-analysis. *Journal of Employment Counseling*, *47*(2), 86–96.

Malle, B. F. (2011). Attribution theories: How people make sense of behavior. *Theories in Social Psychology*, *23*, 72–95.

Marriage, S., & Marriage, K. (2005). Too many sad stories: Clinician stress and coping. *The Canadian Child and Adolescent Psychiatry Review*, *14*(4), 114.

Maslach, C. (2001). What have we learned about burnout and health? *Psychology & Health*, *16*(5), 607–611.

Maslach, C. (2003a). *Burnout: The cost of caring*. Ishk.

Maslach, C. (2003b). Job burnout: New directions in research and intervention. *Current Directions in Psychological Science*, *12*(5), 189–192.

Maslach, C., & Goldberg, J. (1998). Prevention of burnout: New perspectives. *Applied and Preventive Psychology*, *7*(1), 63–74.

Moran, D. (2002). *Introduction to phenomenology*. Oxon: Routledge.

Neff, K. D. (2003). The development and validation of a scale to measure self-compassion. *Self and Identity*, *2*(3), 223–250.

Neff, K. D., & Pommier, E. (2013). The relationship between self-compassion and other-focused concern among college undergraduates, community adults, and practicing meditators. *Self and Identity, 12*(2), 160–176.

Neff, K. D., & Seppälä, E. (2016). Compassion, well-being, and the hypo-egoic self. In *The Oxford handbook of hypo-egoic phenomena* (pp. 189–203). Oxford: Oxford University Press.

Newell, J. M., & MacNeil, G. A. (2010). Professional burnout, vicarious trauma, secondary traumatic stress, and compassion fatigue. *Best Practices in Mental Health, 6*(2), 57–68.

Nielsen, M. B., & Einarsen, S. (2012). Outcomes of exposure to workplace bullying: A meta-analytic review. *Work & Stress, 26*(4), 309–332.

Pack, M. (2014). Vicarious resilience: A multilayered model of stress and trauma. *Affilia, 29*(1), 18–29.

Pakenham, K. I., & Stafford-Brown, J. (2012). Stress in clinical psychology trainees: Current research status and future directions. *Australian Psychologist, 47*(3), 147–155.

Pearlman, L. (1999). Self-care for trauma therapists: Ameliorating vicarious traumatization. In B. H. Stamm (Ed.), *Secondary traumatic stress: Self-care issues for clinicians, researchers, and educators* (2nd ed., pp. 51–64). Lutherville, MD: Sidran Press.

Peterson, C., Semmel, A., Von Baeyer, C., Abramson, L. Y., Metalsky, G. I., & Seligman, M. E. (1982). The attributional style questionnaire. *Cognitive Therapy and Research, 6*(3), 287–299.

Sim, W., Zanardelli, G., Loughran, M. J., Mannarino, M. B., & Hill, C. E. (2016). Thriving, burnout, and coping strategies of early and later career counseling center psychologists in the United States. *Counselling Psychology Quarterly, 29*(4), 382–404.

Skitka, L. J. (1999). Ideological and attributional boundaries on public compassion: Reactions to individuals and communities affected by a natural disaster. *Personality and Social Psychology Bulletin, 25*(7), 793–808.

Slavich, G. M., & Cole, S. W. (2013). The emerging field of human social genomics. *Clinical Psychological Science, 1*(3), 331–348.

Sodeke-Gregson, E. A., Holttum, S., & Billings, J. (2013). Compassion satisfaction, burnout, and secondary traumatic stress in UK therapists who work with adult trauma clients. *European Journal of Psychotraumatology, 4*(1). https://doi.org/10.3402/ejpt.v4i0.21869.

Spreitzer, G., Sutcliffe, K., Dutton, J., Sonenshein, S., & Grant, A. M. (2005). A socially embedded model of thriving at work. *Organization Science, 16*(5), 537–549.

Strauss, C., Taylor, B. L., Gu, J., Kuyken, W., Baer, R., Jones, F., & Cavanagh, K. (2016). What is compassion and how can we measure it? A review of definitions and measures. *Clinical Psychology Review, 47*, 15–27.

Thompson, I., Amatea, E., & Thompson, E. (2014). Personal and contextual predictors of mental health counselors' compassion fatigue and burnout. *Journal of Mental Health Counseling, 36*(1), 58–77.

Zimbardo, P., & Boyd, J. (2008). *The time paradox: The new psychology of time that will change your life*. New York: Simon & Schuster.

CHAPTER 10

Change Outside of the Therapeutic Encounter

Values and beliefs connect with how we practice and how we live. In what ways do they also play into our judgments about diversity, fairness, and equity in society? Do we live in an unfair or unjust society? What is equity, and how does it fit?

THE LOTTERY OF BIRTH

Try the following group activity. You will need special dice available from game stores. The dice needed have many sides and come in colors. Small groups of 10–20 will need 70–140 dice for fantasy board games (in sets of 7). Each set has one die from 4 sides to 10 sides.

Preparation: Organize sets of dice. One set for each player. For each of 10 sets of 7, remove the three die with the most sides. For the remaining ten sets of 7, remove the three die with the fewest sides.

To play: (1) Have participants each select a pack of dice without knowing the contents to make random groups of 3–4. Explain that the number of sides refers to opportunities and the actual numbers, to progress. (2) On a whiteboard construct a chart for each group with names across the top. Record each roll while everyone watches. (3) The first person to reach 250 is the "WINNER!"

© The Author(s) 2019 159
J. D. Brown, *Reflective Practice of Counseling and Psychotherapy in a Diverse Society*, https://doi.org/10.1007/978-3-030-24505-4_10

What is it like to be in your group? How is your group same/different from other groups? What do you like about your group? What don't you like about your group? What do you think about the other groups?

As a counselor, your expertise is a type of power and privilege that we carry in the counseling room. How can we, as counselors, recognize this differential? What might we notice about who comes to see us (who does not) and how they respond to us? What can we do to bridge this difference?

COMMUNITY AND SOCIETY

Consider that within a diverse society, groups have privilege relative to others, and some groups experience more disadvantage than others. The broader social, economic, and political structures reinforce these differences in life opportunities and chances.

Social expectations and judgments exist in the perceptions we hold about members of different groups. Are these expectations and judgments fair? Are these expectations and judgments desirable? Are these expectations and judgments natural? Are they changeable? Do counselors and psychotherapists have a role to play in changing them? What is that role?

How can expectations root in structures that privilege and oppress shift? Consider two fundamental ways to redistribute life opportunities and chances fairly. (1) Make efforts at local, civic, or regional, as well as state or province/territory and national levels. Examples of these appear in case studies at the end of this chapter. (2) Make efforts outside of as well as within the therapeutic encounter. Within the therapeutic encounter, therapists can challenge unhelpful expectations and judgments clients possess. Outside of the therapeutic encounter, therapists can also challenge unhelpful expectations and judgments on behalf of clients through networking and advocacy.

The metaphor of a motorized walkway may be used to represent society (Sue, 2017 citing Tatum, 2001, pp. 11–12). Walking in the direction of the walkway is acting in ways that reinforce dominant patterns. Dominant patterns are evident in classism, racism, ethnocentrism, heterosexism, transphobia, ableism, and ageism. Walking quickly in the walkway direction is active supremacy, while simply walking on the walkway might be termed unintentional supremacy. While non-supremacists do not walk at all, the anti- supremacists walk in the opposite direction or disrupt the walkway itself.

Where do you see yourself on the walkway metaphor? Where do you see your colleagues? Where do you see your clients? What do you do to walk in the opposite direction? What could you do to walk in the opposite direction? What repercussions have you experienced? What repercussions do you anticipate?

Networking and Advocacy

In consideration of the types of activities that counselors and psychotherapists may engage in to improve clients' connections and access to local resources, community building, case networking, outreach, and advocacy are possible.

Group work that has a community-building purpose beyond the therapy itself can be one means by which to reduce isolation and increase social support. There are many examples of such groups in the literature. Friendship groups to women who have limited social connections may improve confidence as well as skills in making friendships, building trust and sense of community (Mentinis, 2015; Newman & Lovell, 1993). Adolescents in an arts-based group were asked to create and present their versions of both the community they lived in and an ideal version (Slayton, 2012). While some groups remain led by a professional facilitator, others might have as a purpose the development of an independent structure that over time reduces and ends the need for a professional to be involved (Jang & Kim, 2012). Such a group may have a specific advocacy view and become a resource for others in the community for support and advice (Reading & Rubin, 2011).

Therapists may choose to become involved in professional networking around a particular issue or more generally, regarding the range of available supports. Supports might include basic needs such as food, clothing, shelter, and agencies or organizations that provide such services. They may also include legal advice, such as accessible or pro-bono services that clients might access. Other potential issues include financial insolvency, human rights, protection for children, law enforcement, relationship violence, spousal support, among many others. In addition to resources that provide a service, self-help or advocacy groups are excellent organizations with which to network. A warm referral where a discussion takes place between the client and therapist about the organization as well as a direct connection with someone at the receiving agency may be especially necessary for some clients who are wary of reaching out on their own.

Case networking works at the interface between clients and their environments (Hepworth, Rooney, Rooney, Strom-Gottfried, & Larsen, 2006). It is one approach to refer to assist a client with a particular need that is met by another organization. Another approach that is less about the acute need and more about the long term is what Fook (1993) calls "radical case networking." In this form, the networking assists a client with the confidence and skill to advocate for self. The main difference is that in radical case networking, the purpose is to change the context that unfairly disadvantages a client, while in typical case networking, the purpose is to find a resource that temporarily meets a need.

Outreach refers to a service offered to a client *where the client is*. While it is much more convenient for a therapist to meet with clients in an office, there are times when it makes sense to meet in another setting. In some types of therapy, for example, exposure therapy, the need to meet outside of the office for practice purposes is part of the therapy itself. In other cases, the need to meet outside of the office might be to get a sense of a person's life in school, at home, or community. Again, a naturalistic setting might be called for by the therapy process itself.

Another potential consideration for engaging in outreach is to make a service more accessible. For example, meeting in a community center where there is a private room and childcare available could be the difference for a busy parent who stays at home and relies on public transportation. There are potential challenges that can interfere, however, such as privacy concerns, absence of professional follow up or security, as well as therapeutically, dual relationship or boundary issues (Rogers & Pilgrim, 2014).

Advocacy *promotes equality, social justice, and social inclusion. It can empower people to speak up for themselves. Advocacy can help people become more aware of their rights, to exercise those rights, and be involved in and influence decisions* (Lee, 2007). Advocacy can be taken up by the therapist or coached and supported in a client. The purpose is to promote fairness on a particular issue for the individual. The willingness and readiness of the client must be present before such efforts are engaged. It is essential to consider one's own needs as a therapist relative to the self-defined needs of a client. For example, a client who feels the influence of the therapist to file a complaint might be feeling the therapists need for the client and not the client's need for self.

SOCIAL ACTION

Social action is an umbrella category for a wide range of efforts for making community change. It is similar to advocacy insofar as the needs or rights of a particular group can be a focus for community change. The multiple forms it takes have a long history. For example, Indigenous leaders organizing to work through treaty negotiation following European contact, years later in many forms of resistance to colonial expansion and control, and today, efforts to promote reconciliation. Other examples include the development of economic cooperatives in Canada's east coast fishing industry, cooperatives, unions. Present-day community action is an extension of efforts undertaken during the Civil Rights movement. Citizen organizing and political activism remain progressive and prominent forces of change in movements such as #metoo and the Women's March.

Approaches to Social Action

The main approaches to social action include locality development, social planning, and social activism (Rothman, 1996). Locality development is a grassroots approach to the development of community members capacity to take action in support of its members. The hallmark of locality approaches to social change is the emphasis on self-help and indigenous leadership. Therapists involved in such efforts as professionals or citizens have little to no role as "experts," but function instead as community members and stakeholders with interest in the community itself, first, and relationships to other communities, second (Green & Haines, 2015).

Social planning is an expert-driven approach to the direction and also methods by which change is most efficiently or expediently pursued. Hallmarks of this approach are the advice of a technical expert in the "problem," methods to arrive at a solution and plan for attainment (Weil, 2014). Therapists involved in such activities may be the expert technician, facilitator, or project manager retained by the community or another body (often, government), to move a process to address an important political issue.

Social activism is an active approach to the inequitable distribution of opportunities and resources among members of a particular group. The hallmark of activism is charismatic leadership using pressure tactics to influence those in power to relinquish controls that lead to unfair treatment. Therapists involved in such activities may be leaders or supporters who declare a position on what they believe is the "right side" of an issue and support the methods used to achieve social change.

Process of Social Action

Social action efforts may take place in steps. These steps do not necessarily occur linearly or simultaneously, may stop as well as regress. The steps include preparation, organization, momentum building, as well as taking and sustaining action. Preparation includes identifying the community, the issue, and a potential solution as well as collecting background information. Organizing is when the individual or small group of constituents reaches out to a broader community to bring in support, formulate priorities, and broaden the effort. Momentum builds through education and social networking.

Additional research may be undertaken on the issue to clarify it further and unify support, with the setting of goals as a desirable outcome. The action stage is often challenging. The support that initiatives often begin with may fade as lives become busy and interest wanes. There may be a renewal of interest by bringing in new members and maintaining lines of communication with all supporters.

SUMMARY

- Social, economic, and political structures create and reinforce the advantage held by members of some groups relative to members of other groups.

- In consideration of the types of activities that counselors and psychotherapists may engage in to improve clients' connections and access to local resources, community building, case networking, outreach, and advocacy is essential.
- Group work that has a community-building purpose beyond the therapy itself can be one means by which to reduce isolation and increase social support.
- Social action is an umbrella category for a wide range of efforts for making community change. It is similar to advocacy insofar as the needs or rights of a particular group can be a focus for community change.

Social Action Case Examples

Social action requires potentially controversial public stances on issues as well as direct action to show support. In the cases that follow, consider your views about the issues, degree of interest, and where you might place your professional or political support.

For each of the cases presented, consider the following questions:

1. What, if anything, is unfair or unjust about the case?
2. Why does it exist? (i.e. what caused it to occur?)
3. What, if anything, can a counselor or psychotherapist do (and not do)? Why?
4. Knowing yourself, your own intersecting identities and experiences with privilege and oppression, what actions are you most personally in favor of and against?
5. What is the best way for you to take action as a (a) citizen, (b) professional, and (c) therapist?

Case 1

A recent video of two young boys in the United States has gone viral. It is of a White boy and his Black friend who has the "same haircut" and therefore, look "the same" to each other. The online discussion has been overwhelmingly positive with multiple news outlets across North America and the UK describing the actions in headlines such as:

White boy asks for the same haircut as Black friend 'to confuse his pre-school teacher.'
Boy has his hair cut like his friend. Now he thinks they can't be told apart.
Two boys, one White and one Black, Get same haircut to trick teacher.
White boy, four, shaves his hair like his Black best friend in adorable hope their teacher wouldn't be able to tell them apart.
White boy asks for same haircut as Black friend so teacher 'won't be able to tell them apart.
Adorable Louisville preschooler thinks a new buzzcut makes him look exactly like his best friend, who's a different race.
Black and White friends try to trick teacher with matching haircuts.

There were also more interpretive headlines.

One little boy's haircut teaches the world about colorblind love.
One haircut, two five-year-old boys and a lesson in racial prejudice.

> What do you think? Do the actions, purpose, or friendship between these boys teach "colorblind love" or "a lesson in racial prejudice"? In what ways does saying "we are all the same" reinforce the status quo? If you were working as a counselor or psychotherapist in the school the boys attended, how would you approach relationships between different races and ethnicities of children?

Case 1 Web Links
White boy Asks for Same Haircut as Black Friend 'To Confuse His Pre-school Teacher'
http://www.telegraph.co.uk/news/2017/03/03/boy-asks-haircut-like-friend-teacher-cant-tell-apart/
Boy Has His Hair Cut Like His Friend. Now He Thinks They Can't Be Told Apart
http://globalnews.ca/news/3285068/jax-reddy-haircut/
One Little Boy's Haircut Teaches the World About Colorblind Love
http://www.kansascity.com/news/nation-world/national/article1360
09253.html.

Case 2

In the fall of 2017, following a series of revelations of sexual impropriety in the American film industry, the hashtag #MeToo was used online by survivors of male to female sexual violence to show support. This phrase, used initially by Tarana Burke on Myspace to empower women of color from disadvantaged communities who were sexually abused, grew exponentially. By identifying as having been assaulted, posts were intended to help those who had experienced sexual violence to know that they were not alone.

In the words of Tarana Burke, *#MeToo is essentially about survivors supporting survivors. And it's really about community healing and community action. Although we can't define with healing looks like for people, we can set the stage and give people the resources to have access to healing. And that means legitimate things like policies and laws that change that* (Business Insider, 2017).

The movement illuminated a magnitude of sexual violence against women worldwide. It made way for legislation to change "cooling off periods" before bringing a complaint forward in the US Congress and drew attention to the practices of Canadian law enforcement about high rates of dismissed sexual assault allegations (Globe & Mail, 2018b).

In a subsequent interview, Burke was quoted as saying *Inherently, having privilege isn't bad…but it's how you use it, and you have to use it in service of other people. Now that I have it, I'm trying to use it responsibly. But if it hadn't come along I would be right here, with my fucking Me Too shirt on, doing workshops and going to rape crisis centers. The work is the work* (*The Guardian*, 2018).

> How do you feel about #MeToo? Has it raised awareness of sexual violence by men against women? Working as a therapist in a higher education context, would you post your support in your office? What would the absence of support communicate to clients?

Case 2 Web Links
Is Inequality Natural?
https://www.psychologytoday.com/us/blog/busting-myths-about-human-nature/201210/is-inequality-natural

The Kind of Racism You Don't Even Know You Have
https://medium.com/@martiesirois/the-kind-of-racism-you-dont-even-know-you-have-44b053cf0c80

Tarana Burke
http://www.businessinsider.com/how-the-metoo-movement-started-where-its-headed-tarana-burke-time-person-of-year-women-2017-12.

Case 3

A recent court case in Saskatchewan, Canada concluded with the acquittal of a non-Indigenous 56-year-old male charged with second-degree murder in the death of a 22-year-old Indigenous male. There was extensive media coverage of the trial and many were deeply troubled by the outcome, including Canada's Prime Minister: *I'm not going to comment on the process that led us to this point today, but I am going to say we have come to this point as a country far too many times…Indigenous people across this country are angry, they're heartbroken, and I know Indigenous and non-Indigenous Canadians alike know that we have to do better* (CTV, 2018).

The process followed for jury selection was particularly problematic. Challenges with the size of the area potential jurors were drawn from were noted. In particular, there were limitations for travel by potential jurors from smaller, northern communities with high proportions of Indigenous peoples. Over 750 individuals were randomly selected and 200 arrived for selection. Legislation allowed for preemptive challenges to potential jury members by legal counsel. There were no Indigenous jury members.

A lawyer following the case offered the view that *because of the racial dynamics, the verdict, whether right or wrong, is incurably tainted. So, the outcome is a disservice not just to Indigenous people who see White justice protecting its own; it is also a disservice to all of us who rely on trials to facilitate closure and healing after tragic controversy by dispensing decisions that earn our respect. We cannot respect this decision because whether the jury engaged in racist thought-processes or not, it looks that way* (Globe and Mail, 2018a).

Do you feel it is fair for an Indigenous person to be convicted by a jury of non-Indigenous peers? Considering the colonial history of Canada and the United States, is this evidence of a systemic problem? Working as a therapist in corrections, how would you incorporate your understanding of race and ethnicity into your networking and therapy efforts?

Case 3 Web Links

'We Have to Do Better': Trudeau Reacts to Gerald Stanley Verdict
https://www.ctvnews.ca/canada/we-have-to-do-better-trudeau-reacts-to-gerald-stanley-verdict-1.3798036

How the Justice System Let Race Taint the Stanley Verdict
https://www.theglobeandmail.com/opinion/how-the-justice-system-let-race-taint-the-stanley-verdict/article37931748

Simply Psychology: Prejudice and Discrimination
https://www.simplypsychology.org/prejudice.html.

Case 4

In Vancouver, British Columbia, the Downtown East Side has been studied extensively because of its status as Canada's poorest postal code (Krausz & Jang, 2015). The community has high rates of mental illness, communicable diseases, and crime (Boyd, Murray, & MacPherson, 2017; Jones, 2015). Two-thirds of the population of about 18,000 live in poverty, and 40% rely on government transfer payments for income (Miewald & Ostry, 2014). The housing stock is old, and many residences are in low-quality single room occupancy hotels (Burnett, 2013). High rates of HIV infections and overdose deaths have led to two public health emergencies in the past 20 years.

Residents with drug use problems in Vancouver's East Side experience multiple challenges. However, local activism has had a significant effect on the resources available (Boyd, Murray, & MacPherson, 2017). Dean Wilson has been a resident for many years and an outspoken advocate for the health needs of drug users (Kerr, Mitra, Kennedy, & McNeil, 2017). In a 2014 interview (Howell) he recalled that his activism *comes from my mother and her real sense of fair play that was drilled into me as a kid. That's, I think, why I got into doing this [activism] because I didn't think that there was a lot of fairness going on with the people who were addicts."

Wilson's activism is well-documented in the film *Fix: The Story of an Addicted City in 2002* where he led the Vancouver Area Network of Drug Users (Damon et al., 2017) to sit-ins at city hall and represented the group in meetings with the mayor, as well as international meetings with law enforcement and healthcare experts.

He made a significant contribution to health care for residents who are drug users earning him the title of Canada's 'most famous junkie'. Efforts such as street health outreach and needle exchange programs as well as supervised injection sites in the area (Jozaghi, 2015). Harm reduction programs have had encouraging results on infection rates and overdose deaths (Jozaghi, Lampkin, & Andresen, 2016).

What role do you see for counseling and psychotherapy in a community with high levels of disadvantage including poverty substance misuse? To what extent are the problems residents face contextual? How much is personal? As a therapist in a community agency would you consider activism and networking to be a priority?

Case 4 Web Links
From Opium to Opioids: A Look at British Columbia's Illicit Drug History
http://toronto.citynews.ca/2017/04/13/from-opium-to-opioids-examining-british-columbias-long-history-with-drugs/

Mental Health: The New Frontier for the Welfare State
https://www.youtube.com/watch?v=fDE45HqcX2A

How Economic Inequality Harms Societies | Richard Wilkinson
https://www.youtube.com/watch?v=cZ7LzE3u7Bw.

Case 5

Controversial public education efforts have garnered a great deal of attention. While anti-discrimination and diversity messages in public institutions have become commonplace and rarely draw attention, this approach certainly does. These advertisements are located in primary and secondary schools in a British Columbia district, on billboards in the city of Saskatoon, Saskatchewan and a university in Oshawa, Ontario.

In British Columbia, "The poster at the centre of the debate features a photo of district superintendent Teresa Downs next to her quote that reads: 'I have unfairly benefited from the colour of my skin. White privilege is not acceptable.'" In her explanation, she notes that "We understand that the discussion of race and privilege can make some people feel uncomfortable,". "But we are also mindful in this district that we cannot have a wholesome conversation about racism without acknowledging that racism results in some groups being privileged."

In Saskatchewan, the billboard "I have to acknowledge my own privilege and racist attitudes," reads the quote on the sign, next to an image of (Jim) Williams. He is also depicted in a campaign video. Although there are four signs, the one depicting Williams appears to have sparked the biggest reaction from residents who feel the sign wrongly implies other Saskatoon residents are racist"

In Ontario, the poster "Becoming aware of privilege should not be viewed as a burden or source of guilt, but rather an opportunity to learn and be responsible so that we may work toward a more just and inclusive world" is placed with another with categories of social privilege defined as "unearned access to social power based on membership in a dominant social group."

Who is the target audience? How important are these messages in confronting White privilege? How do you feel as a White person or person of color about these? How does White privilege play out in your experience? Where do you notice it most? Least? How could it manifest in therapy?

Case 5 Web Links
Poster in B.C. Schools About White Privilege Hits Nerve with Some Parents
https://www.ctvnews.ca/canada/poster-in-b-c-schools-about-white-privilege-hits-nerve-with-some-parents-1.3835619

'I Chose My Words Very Carefully': Face of Anti-Racism Billboard Responds to Backlash
http://www.cbc.ca/news/canada/saskatoon/billboard-racism-saskatoon-response-i-am-the-bridge-1.4190540

Canadian Schools Facing Blowback for 'White Privilege' Awareness Campaigns
http://nationalpost.com/news/canada/canadian-schools-facing-blowback-for-white-privilege-awareness-campaigns.

Case 6

The Women's March as a social movement first took place in January 2017. It was a worldwide movement to advocate for human rights, immigration, healthcare, and environmental reform as well as racial, sexual, and religious equity (Przybyla, 2017). Many rallies were protests against the President of the United States for his positions and his anti-women comments and behavior. The first protest was in Washington, DC and many others across the United States. Supporters from Canada chartered busses to join (Canadian Press, 2017). There were protests in Ottawa and other Canadian cities.

Pink hats will take to the streets again for the second annual Women's March this weekend. Last year's historic march saw millions of demonstrators in 600 cities, on every continent in the world, marching for women's rights and human rights. In the U.S., the 2018 marches are taking place on both days this weekend, with marches in some bigger cities like New York and Washington, D.C., scheduled for Saturday and a new event, Power to the Polls, happening in Las Vegas on Sunday (Langone, 2018).

The Women's March on Washington is a women-led movement bringing together people of all genders, ages, races, cultures, political affiliations, disabilities and backgrounds in our nation's capital on January 21, 2017, to affirm our shared humanity and pronounce our bold message of resistance and self- determination. Recognizing that women have intersecting identities and are therefore impacted by a multitude of social justice and human rights issues, we have outlined a representative vision for a government that is based on the principles of liberty and justice for all. As Dr. King said, "We cannot walk alone. And as we walk, we must make the pledge that we shall always march ahead. We cannot turn back." Our liberation is bound in each other's. (Guiding Vision & Definition of Principles, 2018).

What social problems make the Women's March a necessity? How are these issues relevant to you as a citizen, professional, and in your family roles? How are these issues implicit or explicit in the therapy you provide? Under what circumstances in therapy would you make them explicit? Why?

Case 6 Web Links
Everything You Need to Know About This Year's Women's March http://time.com/5107988/womens-march-2018-las-vegas-chicago-new-york/

Guiding Vision and Definition of Principles
https://static1.squarespace.com/static/584086c7be6594762f5ec56e/
t/587ffb20579fb3554668c111/1484782369253/WMW+Guiding+
Vision+%26+Definition+of+Principles.pdf

Women's March Mission
https://www.womensmarch.com/mission/.

REFERENCES

Boyd, S., Murray, D., & MacPherson, D. (2017). Telling our stories: Heroin-assisted treatment and SNAP activism in the Downtown Eastside of Vancouver. *Harm Reduction Journal, 14*(1), 27.

Burnett, K. (2013). Commodifying poverty: Gentrification and consumption in Vancouver's Downtown Eastside. *Urban Geography, 35*(2), 157–176.

Business Insider. (2017). Retrieved from www.businessinsider.com/how-the-metoo-movement-started-where-its-headed-tarana-burke-time-person-of-year-women-2017–12.

Canadian Press. (2017). *Thousands across Canada rally in support of Women's March on Washington.* Retrieved from https://www.theglobeandmail.com/news/national/events-organized-across-canada-to-support-washington-womens-march/article33696331/.

CTV. (2018). 'We have to do better': Trudeau reacts to Gerald Stanley verdict. Retrieved from https://www.ctvnews.ca/canada/we-have-to-do-better-trudeau-reacts-to-gerald-stanley-verdict-1.3798036.

Damon, W., Callon, C., Wiebe, L., Small, W., Kerr, T., & McNeil, R. (2017). Community-based participatory research in a heavily researched inner city neighbourhood: Perspectives of people who use drugs on their experiences as peer researchers. *Social Science and Medicine, 176,* 85–92.

Fook, J. (1993). *Radical casework: A theory of practice.* St Leonards, NSW, Australia: Allen & Unwin.

Globe and Mail. (2018a). *How the justice system let race taint the Stanley verdict.* Retrieved from https://www.theglobeandmail.com/opinion/how-the-justice-system-let-race-taint-the-stanley-verdict/article37931748/.

Globe and Mail. (2018b). Retrieved from www.theglobeandmail.com/news/investigations/unfounded-37272-sexual-assault-cases-being-reviewed-402-unfounded-cases-reopened-so-far/article37245525/.

Green, G. P., & Haines, A. (2015). *Asset building & community development.* Los Angeles: Sage.

Hepworth, D. H., Rooney, R. H., Rooney, G. D., Strom-Gottfried, K., & Larson, J. (2006). *Direct social work practice: Theory and skills.* Belmont, CA: Cengage Learning.

Jang, M., & Kim, Y. H. (2012). The effect of group sandplay therapy on the social anxiety, loneliness and self-expression of migrant women in international marriages in South Korea. *The Arts in Psychotherapy, 39*(1), 38–41.

Jones, A. A. (2015). Mental illness and significant cognitive impairment among marginalized adults in Vancouver's Downtown Eastside. *Addiction, 110*(10), 1605–1614.

Jozaghi, E. (2015). *The role of peer drug users' social networks and harm reduction programs in changing the dynamics of life for people who use drugs in the downtown eastside of Vancouver, Canada* (Doctoral dissertation). Arts and Social Sciences.

Jozaghi, E., Lampkin, H., & Andresen, M. A. (2016). Peer-engagement and its role in reducing the risky behavior among crack and methamphetamine smokers of the Downtown Eastside community of Vancouver, Canada. *Harm Reduction Journal, 13*(1), 19.

Kerr, T., Mitra, S., Kennedy, M. C., & McNeil, R. (2017). Supervised injection facilities in Canada: Past, present, and future. *Harm Reduction Journal, 14*(1), 28.

Krausz, M., & Jang, K. (2015). Lessons from the creation of Canada's poorest postal code. *The Lancet Psychiatry, 2*(3), e5.

Lee, S. (2007). *Making decisions: The independent mental capacity advocacy service.* London, UK: Mental Capacity Implementation Program.

Mentinis, M. (2015). Friendship: Towards a radical grammar of relating. *Theory & Psychology, 25*(1), 63–79.

Miewald, C., & Ostry, A. (2014). A warm meal and a bed: Intersections of housing and food security in Vancouver's Downtown Eastside. *Housing Studies, 29*(6), 709–729.

Newman, J. A., & Lovell, M. (1993). A description of a supervisory group for group counselors. *Counselor Education and Supervision, 33*, 22–31.

Przybyla, H. (2017). *Women's march an 'entry point' for a new activist wave.* Retrieved from https://www.usatoday.com/story/news/politics/2017/01/05/womens-march-searches-themes-amid-concern-trump-gop-congress/96199000/.

Reading, R., & Rubin, L. R. (2011). Advocacy and empowerment: Group therapy for LGBT asylum seekers. *Traumatology, 17*(2), 86–98.

Rogers, A., & Pilgrim, D. (2014). *A sociology of mental health and illness.* London: McGraw-Hill Education.

Rothman, J. (1996). The interweaving of community intervention approaches. *Journal of Community Practice, 3*(3–4), 69–99.

Slayton, S. C. (2012). Building community as social action: An art therapy group with adolescent males. *The Arts in Psychotherapy, 39*(3), 179–185.

Sue, D. W. (2017). The challenges of becoming a White Ally. *The Counseling Psychologist*, 45(5), 706–716.

Tatum, B. D. (2001). Defining racism: Can we talk. In P. S. Rothenberg (Ed.), *Race, Class, and Gender in the United States: An integrated Study* (pp. 100, 107). New York: Worth Publishers.

The Guardian. (2018). Retrieved from www.theguardian.com/world/2018/jan/15/me-too-founder-tarana-burke-women-sexual-assault.

Weil, M. (2014). *Community practice: Conceptual models*. New York: Routledge.

INDEX

© The Editor(s) (if applicable) and The Author(s) 2019
J. D. Brown, *Reflective Practice of Counseling and Psychotherapy
in a Diverse Society*, https://doi.org/10.1007/978-3-030-24505-4